CW01456457

THE VASECTOMY DIARIES

A Tale of Hard Decisions, Empty Emissions, and Tiny Incisions

By Rodney Lacroix

Dedication

This book is dedicated to the millions of my sperm who will never find a home and my two nuts who gave up their perfect, globular glory to make sure I will never seed another pasture ever again.

I am also dedicating this to all the men who are thinking of undergoing the procedure or who have already had it done.

We are legion.

We are a sterile, scarred legion.

Never forget that.

Table of Contents

Kids: Because every so often, you need a reminder why your vasectomy was a great idea.

Introduction

Hi there.

My name is Rodney Lacroix and, for those of you who don't know me, I am an author and comedian. I have written several books poking fun at an array of different things, ranging from parenting to romance to a wonderful tale about crapping my pants on a bicycle.

However, in these very pages you hold, I'm going to talk to you about something that no one should joke about:

Balls.

That's right. Scrotum.

The Testicle Twins.

Lefty and Righty.

Scrotes McGotes.

Balls.

This book is about balls.

For guys, it's about those two (or three, depending on how close you live to a nuclear power plant) gross dangly sacks of wrinkly dough bobbling around down between their legs like hideous Christmas ornaments. They are inconveniently placed and somehow always in the way.

They are overly tender, and not just in the way they cry while watching *Beaches*. Sitting on them will make you scream. If you get hit in them, even slightly, any activity you are participating in must be put on hold for a minimum of ten minutes while you writhe around in agony.

During this time, women are yelling things like, "Suck it up," while other guys are feeling sympathy pains, standing around cradling their own nads, and consoling each other.

When it's warm or humid, they glue themselves to the inside of your thigh. This is uncomfortable and forces you to do this weird squat-stretch like a Sumo wrestler, hoping that your legs open enough for your sticky sacks to peel themselves off and go back to their regular dangly position.

When it's cold out, they pack their bags and head for a warmer climate. Oftentimes, they won't even send you a postcard or tell you when they're coming back.

Then there are the times you get bored and just fiddle with them. You roll them around like Ben Wa balls or wrap them up and over your penis to make your dick look like Mickey Mouse.

We've all done it. Don't pretend you don't Mickey Mouse your privates.

Men, this is also about what to expect when you're expecting to have those two little blobs carved up and cauterized so you don't make any more babies. It is about the process of deciding between your nuts going under a scalpel or continuing with a full clip in your Magnum and risk having another child that will torment you and make you bald.

Spoiler alert: taking a scalpel to the slappers is totally worth it.

Ladies, for you this book is about understanding the pain and struggle of our choice in taking one for the team. Or two for the team, depending on how you look at it. It is for you to understand what *we* go through so *you* don't have to go through another childbirth. It's also so we don't have to hear you bitch about going through another childbirth. Men are selfish.

I hope you enjoy reading this. If you are considering a vasectomy, I hope it gives you a little insight into the entire process. If you've already had a vasectomy, I hope you find something in here that you can relate to and find some joy in reliving the entire experience even though I use words like "searing" and "needle" and "Deflategate," which may actually trigger some Vietnam-type flashbacks in a few of you.

Maybe we should start a support group.

Ladies, we all know how much you enjoy seeing men suffer so this should be hysterical for you.

In any case, male or female, I hope you enjoy the book. In fact, feel free to go nuts.

Nuts.

Man. I really miss those guys.

Chapter 1

The Decision for an Incision

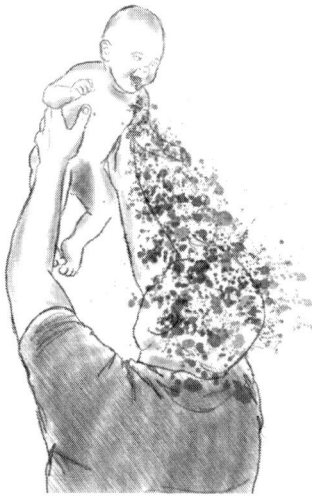

My daughter got syrup on her socks and is now trying to stick them on my bedroom wall. Things like this are why vasectomies exist.

Day 1

Well, hello Diary.

I have never fancied myself as a "diary writer" or "journal keeper" but the fact that I just used the word "fancied" seems to contradict that notion. Yet, here I am, frantically typing away in this thing like a crazy person. Scratch that. I am typing along like a crazy *sexy* person.

This diary also serves as an acknowledgment of my narcissism.

I decided to start writing this after having an epiphany earlier today. Normally, any epiphany I have is followed shortly by some sort of sandwich, because most of my great ideas involve making lunch. However, today an enlightening realization happened as I stood smack-dab in the middle of a Chuck E. Cheese while attending my daughter's seventh birthday party:

I hate children.

Okay. Maybe "hate" is a strong word. *I strongly dislike* children.

Not my children, mind you. I like *my* kids.

It's other people's children I dislike. Immensely.

What you need to know, Diary, is that I have two kids. Payton has just turned seven and my son, Cameron, is only three. The four-year difference between their ages is directly related to Payton driving me and my wife absolutely batshit crazy for the first three years of her life.

Payton was born colicky and either cried or screamed constantly for 24 hours a day right up until about the age of two. This was a great transition for her to slide directly into the 'terrible twos' which basically entails every parent yelling "NO NO NO NO" or "STOP IT" or "SOMEONE

3

PLEASE KILL ME" from the moment children wake up to when they finally fall asleep three hours past their bedtime after the 16th time they've gotten out of bed.

I have not slept in seven years.

The first three years were so hard on us that we did not even *consider* discussing having another child. In fact, there were several times I applied to be a nun but it turns out that men can't be nuns, which seems like some sort of bullshit to me. Someday there will be a man-nun and he will be a hero to all, like Rosa Parks or the first person to put sauerkraut on a corned beef sandwich. *OHMYGOD I hope the man-nun is named "Reuben."* Actually, I think Reuben is a Jewish name so maybe that is not possible unless he converts first.

Dear Diary: I have adult Attention Deficit Disorder, as an FYI.

Eventually, though, we figured that I was getting too old to be a new dad. I was 34 years old in 2002 and had a diet that consisted primarily of squirt-cheese in a can, so I was probably running out of time to have another kid before I died or my sperm dried up and turned to dust. In addition, I have no idea how the reproductive system works.

Cameron showed up in 2003 and was the opposite of Payton. This means he was quiet. When you parent a colicky child, having a quiet one is just as disconcerting. We would be waking up in the middle of the night all panicky like "WHY ISN'T HE SCREAMING OHMYGOD WE MUST CHECK ON HIM" and then bolt out of our bed but he'd just be asleep. This went on for about six months until we realized some kids actually do not scream constantly.

Well, we *thought* some kids do not scream constantly.

That brings me back to the birthday party at Chuck E. Cheese.

I stood there today amidst a sea of glassy-eyed, sugared-up children eating bad pizza while chewing with their mouths open and surveyed the situation. Some of the kids were playing games, some were dragging their moms around and others were shooting me nasty looks because I was hogging up the attention of *their* moms by showing them how I could make my pecs dance to the A-B-C song.

Always a crowd pleaser, that one.

It was on or around the third time my temple split open from the pressure of the headache caused by the 132-decibel level of the beeps, blorts, yells, and screams that the gum-stained ceiling of Chuck E. Cheese opened up and heavenly rays shone down upon me. I became instantly enlightened.

I must kill my sperm.

Kids are evil.

This is Hell.

I already have two kids, a boy and a girl. It is the perfect balance of children. It's like an even match of good versus evil, love versus hate, or Simon versus Garfunkel. The two cancel each other out. Add a third munchkin into the mix and it could send my world into a tailspin.

I also have not been on a vacation since the year 2000, unless you count that time I was allowed to go to the drug store alone to get more aspirin for our constant migraines. Furthermore, I do not want to be faced with the prospect of cleaning up a diaper at the age of 40, unless it is my own. God that sounds gross. Why did I even go there? My brain is mush. This is what children do to us.

So there, right there, I decided.

It was time for a vasectomy.

I searched the Chuck E. Cheese for my wife and finally found her trying to fish my son out of a ball pit that probably had more germs in it than the cold storage room at the CDC. I yelled to her above the tinnitus-inducing din, because there was no way I was coming anywhere near her. Elbows-deep in a sea of plastic balls and toddlers, she had most likely been infected with 36 strains of some yet-undiscovered child-borne illness.

"HEY!" I shouted, "I THINK I SHOULD-"

"YOU SHOULD GET A VASECTOMY" she interjected and I could clearly see she was already getting some sort of rash ohmygod she is going to die because of this ball pit.

Okay then. I guess I will be getting a vasectomy.

Day 2

I have been rethinking my decision to get a vasectomy.

Why? Because I had a horrible nightmare last night.

In this nightmare, I woke up on an operating table in a large, sterile operating room. I was alone except for someone in scrubs standing in the corner.

"Excuse me?" I said.

There was no reply.

I tried to get up off the table but was powerless to do so. When I looked to see what was holding me down, there were four little babies sitting on my wrists and ankles. It was creepy and I tried to scream but the only sound that came out was a duck call. I quacked and quacked and all it did was make the baby-restraints giggle and that made me giggle which, of course, came out as more duck quacks. It got nuts in there pretty fast with all the quacking and baby-giggling, let me tell you.

"ARE YOU READY?" came the voice from the corner.

I turned my head and looked at the person walking towards me.

I quack-gasped, horrified.

The babies giggled because, seriously, it was this cute little qua-

"I SAID ARE YOU READY?"

I stopped laughing and looked at the man approaching.

It was Johnny Depp completely in character as Edward Scissorhands.

I tried to yell NOOOOOOOOOOO but before I could he was already doing that weird shrubbery-shredding thing with his giant scissor hands and bits of my pubes were flying all over the place and OHMYGOD ONE GOT IN MY MOUTH ACCKKKK ACCCCCKKKKKKK NO WONDER WOMEN DON'T LIKE GOING DOWN THERE ACCKKKKKK but the pubes kept-a-flyin' and things started to get hazy.

I woke up from the nightmare, soaked in sweat and screaming.

"QUAAAACCCKK!"

My wife woke with a jolt. "What the fuck was that?" she asked.

"I had a nightmare," I said. "I don't think I want to go through with the vasectomy."

"Yes, you do," she said. "Goodnight. Stop quacking."

Well, then. I guess that's settled.

Day 4

Sorry I haven't written in a couple of days, but I have been making some phone calls about getting this vasectomy.

It turns out that your regular doctor does not do this procedure. This is a good thing for me because my doctor is a woman and I do not want her cutting my testicles open. I have no idea if maybe she has had some bad experience with a dude and now she is all, like, I MUST MAKE MEN PAY and next thing I know I am having wiener-reattachment surgery and she's serving 10 years in an upscale prison with 30 rough pencil sketches she drew of my detached winky hanging on her cell walls. Some of the drawings show him in different outfits and action scenes, including a stunningly realistic depiction of my Mr. Wiggly crossing the Delaware.

It's creepy, but it is nice to know she is still thinking of me while in the clink.

So I called a urologist today. The term "urologist" is derived from the Greek "urolog" meaning "your log area" and the suffix "ist" which translates to, "I guess." I'd look this up but I'm almost positive that's correct. However, I think a better name for the doctor who works on your penis would be like "Dicktor" – a dick doctor.

Then I am informed by the medical terrorist on the phone that a vasectomy is not surgery for your penis at all, but is all about a procedure on your balls. The call was already proving to be an enlightening experience. It also proved that I really paid zero attention in Health Class back in middle school, holy shit, because I had no idea how my own body even worked and I have owned it for most of my life.

The urologist I am going to is actually a male doctor. I'm not sure why I feel more comfortable showing my jumble-giblets to a man than a woman, but maybe I think that is a topic for another diary. It's not like I'm uncomfortable taking everything out in front of a woman, I'm just thinking that when the guy laughs it won't hurt my feelings as much.

Anyway, the receptionist at the urology place told me I needed to schedule two visits.

"One for each ball?" I asked.

There was a minute or so of dead silence after that.

Turns out that the first visit is just a consultation. The doctor examines you, sits you down, tells you what to expect and then probably calls an ambulance for you when you pass out. The second visit is the actual procedure where they proceed to murder your junk.

My first consultation visit is in three days. I swear to God if Johnny Depp visits me again between now and then I am suggesting my wife just stay on the pill forever and ever or until her uterus dries out, whichever comes first.

Day 5

No new ball news today other than I did not have any nightmares about the procedure.

I did, though, have a dream that involved Mr. Bean and the fat kid from the movie *SuperBad* and a small bank heist but the getaway car was a mechanical ostrich. I think I really need to stop eating sugary cereals after 9 PM.

I did call my insurance company and was told that my vasectomy will be covered, as will be the pain pills. This is the first time I've thought about pain. I'm not a fan of pain. Pain is painful. That is probably why they call it pain.

> **Guy #1:** This wound is painful.

> **Guy #2:** We should call what you are feeling, "pain."

> **Guy #1:** I will draw up the legal documents to have this copyrighted.

Sadly, it was never copyrighted and the guy with the wound and his buddy died penniless on the streets of Baltimore, probably.

I am no stranger to pain. I have had plenty of surgeries and stuff done on my shoulders and back because I'm apparently made of balsa wood. After every surgery, I get a prescription for Vicodin or something like that, which I thoroughly enjoy because it numbs my emotions better than the holidays. It also gives me an excuse to not wash dishes because when I'm on painkillers I tend to start throwing them, thinking they're Frisbees. After I destroyed the third set of our wedding china, I was barred from entering the kitchen whenever I took a pill.

So many benefits to prescription meds.

However, the thought of having nut pain never really crossed my mind. Now that I think about it, I know I have seen shows and movies where guys have to put bags of peas on their crotch after getting a vasectomy. We are not huge on vegetables in this house so I'm hoping I can just hold a frozen microwaveable burrito there and it will have the same effect.

Great. Now I want a burrito.

BRB

Day 6

The burrito was delicious.

Tomorrow is the big day of my consultation, so I spent the day in the shower really scrubbing up my joy jungle. I do not want to pull my pants down in front of the doctor and have it be like Pig-Pen from Charlie Brown, with a big dust cloud surrounding my penis and little scratches and dirt marks on his face.

Not that my penis has a face.

I washed the marker off so it's gone now.

I used a facecloth so I know it is all super clean down there and I even used some powder. I have never used powder before so I had absolutely NO idea how much to use. It turns out that a teeny tiny bit of powder goes a really long way. I wish I had known that before I did it because I took a handful and kind of *WHAPPED* it on using my open palm, which hurt a little bit. When the powder-dust cleared, it looked like my penis had been replaced by a tiny cyclops-mime.

Of course, I then had to put him in a little black and white outfit and made him do that "I'm trapped in a box" routine, which is funny when you think about a penis being trapped in a box (wink). So another hour after cleaning all the powder out from my nooks and crannies, I think I'm all ready to go.

Ugh. I am so nervous I feel like throwing up last night's burrito.

Day 7

7:00 AM

IT'S CONSULTATION DAY.

I leave for the urologist's office in about an hour, so I figured I would check in and wish myself luck here. Now this seems stupid. I am going to look back on this and go, "Oh, look, I wished myself luck" instead of kissing my kids goodbye because what if I die during this consultation? I don't want the last words to my son to be "ATOMIC WEDGIE" if I croak. You never know what is going to happen.

Let's say I drop my pants and I'm standing there and the doctor is, like, "Where the hell are your genitals?" so I bend down to show him the last spot I actually saw the little guys hiding. Meanwhile, the doctor, at the very same moment I am bending down, stands up and we bump noggins. Then I get a brain aneurysm and die on the spot with my pants down and then the nurses come in and take pictures posing with my naked corpse. This will be my fifteen minutes of fame because this footage will go viral on YouTube and appear on TMZ.

Great. I am going to die. I am going to die while having a vasectomy consultation. Well, I guess that's another way to ensure I won't have any more kids.

Check in with you guys later.

I hope it's not via YouTube.

14

6:45 PM

Okay. I had the consultation but there is *so much* to talk about that I am going to push it off until tomorrow. In addition, I did not die.

OR DID I?

This could actually be writing from the grave. Oooooooh suddenly this diary has become spooky. Perhaps this diary is actually written by M. Night Shyamalan and the twist at the end is that I've been dead this entire time and whoever is reading this is the one getting the vasectomy. Now you'll have to go re-read this thing to see if I've been dropping clues from the very beginning. I may go back later and add in an appearance on the first page by Haley Joel Osment saying, "I see dead sperm," just for effect.

Back to the consultation.

I did not die but I do have a lot to talk about. One of these things is that the doctor's assistant was the one who did the actual consultation and – dramatic pause - IT WAS A WOMAN ASSISTANT.

[extreme close-up of my face as Dun-dun-DUUUUUUUUUN sound plays]

A woman in charge of scrutinizing my nether region. It was my worst fear coming true.

Well, not my worst, worst fear. My worst fears are the Johnny Depp/Edward Scissorhands scenario and dying pant-less on the examination room floor from trauma caused by an inadvertent doctor/patient head-butt. Having a woman giving me my vasectomy consultation, though, is definitely a solid third.

Chapter 2

The Consultation

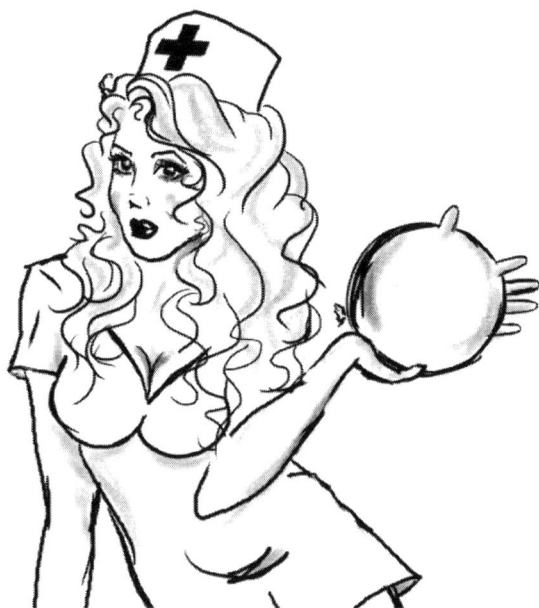

Just scored a new toaster by using my Reward Card from my urologist.

I've been going back once a week to make sure my vasectomy has stuck.

Of Chicken Hats and Alien Heads

Okay, I have some time so I am going to do the best recap I can of yesterday's consultation. I'm giving the consultation its own section in this diary because there is a lot of information to talk about. Also, my wife wanted to go to the mall so I brought the diary with me. Usually, I am just left to die while I wait outside of a JC Penney store with the other men who were dragged shopping, but this gives me something to kill the time. She said she needed to get a new sweater so I figure I have at least 16 hours of writing time right now.

Here goes.

I am almost over my embarrassment of the urologist's female assistant doing the consultation and not the actual doctor. Almost. Every time I think of a strange woman looking at Captain Schlong and his Two Apprentices and I have not paid her for the privilege, it makes me feel a little cheap.

As I sat in the waiting area of the office, I found a number of pamphlets to read. Some were about venereal diseases and stuff and there was one about vasectomies. I always avoid reading venereal disease pamphlets because all they do is make me 99.9% sure I have some sort of herpes because all the risk factors they list out are basically what I consider a fun Tuesday night. I am also scared I may open one and see my own picture in there with "THE INNOCENT FACE OF SYPHILIS" in bold letters as the caption.

I also looked around and saw a bunch of women in the waiting room. I did not know if they were there for the recovery of their man getting a vasectomy, to cheer on the doctors, or were maybe there for their own penis surgeries. There was also the chance that they were just really ugly guys, I had no idea.

Me [leaning toward the man next to me]: What's with all the women here?

Guy: What?

Me: Do you think they have penises too?

Guy: The fuck?

Me: *Well, we're at a urologist. Think they've got* [puts hand down pants and sticks thumb out zipper]

Guy: Dude. It's a UROLOGIST. It's a urinary tract doctor. All people have that.

Me: Hahahaha you're funny. Okay. Go back to your herpes pamphlet, Mr. Herpes.

I opened my own vasectomy pamphlet and started reading about what was going to happen during the consultation. Turns out it's where they tell you all about the procedure, discuss your state of mind, talk about the state of your penis, funny names for your testicles (this was not in the pamphlet but I assumed the omission was just a printing error) and reversibility of the procedure.

Reversibility?

Personally, I am not sure who would want to reverse this. I was nervous enough thinking about Vlad the Executioner with the giant battle-axe lopping off my giblets. Why would you want to go BACK to the scene of the crime after having that done?

Jackass: Hey doc, remember how you cut open my balls and severed a piece of my anatomy?

Doctor: Of course. I'm still getting money from your HMO for it.

Jackass: Well, I have decided that I no longer enjoy sleep, and want another child. I also enjoy the feeling of having stitches on my nutsack. Can you violently cut into them again?

Doctor: Of course I can. Where's your insurance card?

I was about three minutes into creating this elaborate conversation in my head when I was finally called to come in for the consultation. I walked into an eerily quiet, blue room, and sat on a typical patient table that was covered in light blue vinyl and had that giant roll of toilet paper covering it.

I have never understood that roll of paper on the patient tables. Does it have special germ-absorbing power? Let's say a person with leprosy comes in and sits down on the paper and then they roll the paper away and I come and sit down on the next section of paper. Is there no leprosy still floating in the air? Isn't it possible that a leprosy particle crawled over to the section of the paper I'm sitting on at this very moment? WebMD has no answers for this and also they have blacklisted me from their site. I've asked Siri a number of times about this as well and now she is no longer speaking to me.

Not wanting leprosy, I jumped down from the table and then put on some rubber gloves and wiped any potential leper-germs off the seat of my jeans. Then I took the gloves off, got another one out of the bin and made myself an inflatable chicken head. Aside from the potential for contracting an incurable disease from table-paper, this consultation was going much better than I thought it would.

I started looking around and noticed that the walls were adorned with pictures of aliens. One of the aliens had a really long nose like an aardvark and another resembled Shrek, except he had no facial features and at the top of his ears were two balloons. Upon further examination, I realized I was looking at pictures of the male and female reproductive systems. It is here that I need to make a note to myself to find a copy of these diagrams because I honestly thought "urethra" was what miners yelled when they found gold.

It only took me a few seconds to realize I was going to be in trouble. According to these diagrams, my penis was supposed to be three feet long. The front view of the male anatomy looked like an x-ray of Squidward from *Spongebob Squarepants*. I mean, kudos to the guy who was a model for this poster, but if this diagram is anatomically correct then I got really screwed in the endowment department. Honestly, I could probably have sex with this guy's urethra. HA. I am actually proud of myself for using that word in the correct context right now.

Then the doctor's assistant came in.

Braveheart Torture and the Art of Shaving

"OH NO," I thought. "IT IS A WOMAN."

And oh sonofabitch she was ridiculously hot.

Now, as erotic as the prospect of having a hot woman discussing your genitalia in detail sounds, it is not so pleasant when she is about to start talking about carving them up like miniature holiday hams. I mean, even Lorena Bobbitt was hot, but I do not think John would have been able to get it up if she slinked up to him in bed that night holding a knife sharpener and singing *Three Blind Mice*.

This is why I did not have a boner during the appointment. Additionally, it was really really cold in the room, which I think they do for comedic effect.

> **Assistant:** Okay, let's see what we are working with here. *[raises johnnie]*

> **Me:** [looking like Buffalo Bill in Silence of the Lambs when he tucks everything under]

> **Assistant:** Ummm. Where is everything? *[looks at chart]* You are a male, right?

> **Me:** It is like 30 degrees in here. All my bits are back in my abdomen trying to comfort each other and telling ghost stories by a campfire about a crazed urologist armed with a scalpel.

While she was admiring the amazing job I did on my rubber-glove chicken head (it really was spectacular), I took the opportunity to blow warm air on my hands and stuff them into my crotch. It ended up being a successful effort in getting my genitalia heated up enough to where they felt comfortable dropping back down from my belly.

She turned away from my chicken and asked me to hop back up on the examination table. I climbed upon the seat and "protective" paper, figuring that with a penis one-quarter the size of a normal one based on these diagrams, a bout of leprosy was the least of my worries.

She wheeled herself over to the desk on the far side of the room and came back holding a plastic model of a man's reproductive system. The only time I have ever seen one of these models in person was back when I went to a gay bar in Boston in the late '80s and they had them as table centerpieces.

She took the top of the plastic penis off to display the inner workings of the thing. This caused me to scream a little, which I think is just an automatic reaction that happens when you see someone forcibly pull apart genitals. The fact that she went "BWAHAHAHAHAHA TAKE THAT, JOHN, I HOPE YOU'RE HAPPY WITH YOUR UGLY NEW WHORE" while doing it did not help calm my fears any, either.

She proceeded to use a shiny silver pen as a pointer, outlining the procedure that was going to happen. I'm not sure why she used the pen instead of just pointing things out with her finger. In hindsight, it was probably because I whispered, "Oh, yeah, touch it" under my breath every time she approached the plastic model with her hand.

I assume she spoke some big words but lost me when she said the term, "vas deferens." Saying "vas deferens" made me think of Van Halen, and suddenly she sounded like Charlie Brown's teacher as I drifted off and imagined my balls singing "Jump." My left testicle was Dangly Lee Roth and my right one was Eddie Vas Deferens and I started giggling because Dangly tried to stuff himself into Spandex pants and it really wasn't working for him.

"Any questions?" the doctor's assistant asked.

"Yes," I replied. "Can you please repeat everything because…uhh…never mind you don't want to know."

She looked at me blankly and then sighed which, honestly, I get a lot as a typical response. She went over the entire procedure for me again. Thinking back now, I really wish I'd have just said "Oh, yes, I understand everything," and then continued to be oblivious to the procedure and just keep listening to Vas Deferens in my head.

Now I have to add a disclaimer for the remainder of this section because at this point things get pretty graphic. Here goes:

Dear Diary: Please note that if there are stains on this page it's just from my vomit by retelling this procedure.

Essentially, the doctor will numb my chestnuts. This is done with a needle and, sadly, not through Swedish massage performed by several hot Asian women with secret, ancient herbs. Science is stupid.

No, they numb it with A NEEDLE TO MY BALLS.

[insert Psycho shower music here]

I want to die just thinking about it.

I do not like needles. The thought of just getting a needle in my arm gets me all panicky and sweaty and if my mom isn't around, I will usually start crying. Flu shots are a lot of fun for the technician at CVS, let me tell you.

These needles, though, go right into the testicles like William Tell shooting an apple except the apple is between your legs, there are two of them, and also they feel extreme pain. On a related note, my mother declined my requests to hold my hand for this.

Then a second needle goes into the other one. This is why I am jealous of men who only have one nut. A one-nut vasectomy only requires one needle. Two nuts? Two shots. It's as if we are being punished for having proper anatomy. Such bullshit.

Once they are numbed up, the doctor goes in with the scalpel.

At this point in the conversation, I requested a water break. The receptionist, who had come in to see what all the sobbing was about, granted this.

I was able to compose myself after a few short hours and the assistant proceeded with outlining the procedure. The doctor will make a small incision in each testicle, reach in with a medieval instrument of torture and pull out a tube called a "vas deferens." This is the term that sent me daydreaming earlier, but now I had no interest in getting lost in thought again because now my image of Dangly Lee Roth had him standing on stage with a needle jammed into his skull and his face was split open.

Based on how this was being described, I am positive this was the procedure being done to William Wallace at the end of *Braveheart*. Back then, a vasectomy was called "purification by pain."

Now that the vas deferens is exposed, the doctor snips it and then either ties it like the knot I made in my glove-chicken or cauterizes it. Yes, the word "cauterize" and "testicles" was used in the same sentence. Right about here, the receptionist came back in to ask me to please stop crying because patients in the lobby were starting to leave.

> **Assistant:** So, *now* do you have any questions?

> **Me:** No. I used to wonder about the existence of God but now I know he doesn't exist so I have no further questions, your Honor.

I was catatonic at this point and just wanted to leave. I did not want to undergo this procedure anymore. I did not want to be carved up and pierced and disemboweled and burned alive. I did not want a free Scotland if it meant I was going to be in this much agony. I really didn't know how this could get much worse.

Then she told me to lie down on the table as she lifted the hospital gown to take a close-up look at Mr. Wiggly and the Twins so there was my answer.

Assistant: WHOA.

Wait.

Whoa?

Did she just say "Whoa?"

Was it a good "whoa" or a bad "whoa?" What kind of medical professional says "whoa?" OH GREAT NOW ALL I CAN THINK ABOUT IS JOEY LAWRENCE.

Me: Excuse me?

Assistant: Okay. Well, one thing you will need to do before the procedure is shave this entire area.

SHAVE MY AREA?!?!

I was born in 1968. I grew up in the 1970s. I started watching porn back in the mid-to-late '80s. All the porn guys had fantastic mustaches and body hair and everyone's crotch sported an afro. This was what I knew to be the norm.

I have heard rumors of men who shaved their balls. However, the rumors were always sparse and never substantiated. There was even a new term for it floating around:

"Manscaping," they called it.

I assumed manscaping solely existed in secret circles and was some sort of ritual only performed by the Illuminati and people in California named "Chad." I have always been an avid gym-goer and have never seen a male's shaved privates. Not that I've tried to look at other men's crotches. Sometimes I look by accident. One exception is if the man in the locker room is smaller than me, then I will look on purpose because males who are smaller than me are rare. It's really just a look simply for comparison. You know, I really wish I could just stop talking sometimes.

Me: Shave? Shave what? What do I have to shave?

Assistant: All of it.

I sat up a little bit to see what she was talking about. She was gesturing her hands in a big circle when she said "all of it," like she was a paper company executive looking over a topographical map of the rainforest and telling her bulldozer guys how much needed to be cleared out.

"All of it," she said. "We need all this cleared out."

I looked down at my waist and could see my tiny little mushroom head barely poking out of a sea of poofy brown curly-qs. Okay. I guess I could see her point. My crotch looked like a helicopter view of Bob Ross.

Maybe I *did* let this grow a little out of hand. To stress this point, two small birds suddenly emerged and flew out of my groin.

Me: Can I leave just one for old time's sake? I will name him "Alfalfa."

Assistant:

Me: I will take that as a "no."

Then she started to talk about the post-procedure.

This woman had seriously started taking all the fun out of my day. Luckily, I had my inflated latex-glove chicken head — that I decided to name "Alfalfa" after the doctor's assistant shot my idea down — to lighten my mood. She could make me lose my pubes, but she couldn't make me lose my sense of humor.

Although based on her post-procedure talk, she certainly wasn't going to stop trying.

Hallucinations, Human Hair Dryers, and Hairy Palms

I was ready for this consultation to be over. I am not sure what else she could have gone through at this point to make me feel worse other than singing Sarah McLachlan songs while showing me slides of homeless dogs.

I think she may have just been keeping me around a little longer for the company, what with my sweet glove-chicken making skills and whatnot. You cannot deny the allure of a man who can properly inflate a latex glove. I tell myself this in the mirror every morning.

> **Assistant:** Okay, so now we will talk about what happens after the procedure.

Whatever. I bet she still loved my glove-chicken.

She began to discuss what would happen AFTER everything was shaved, snipped, sealed, and burned. I assumed that this simply entailed being in a wheelchair for three months and having some sort of physical therapy where I would need to work the strength back up in my testicles. I pictured it like a montage of Rocky working out, but instead of Sylvester Stallone, it's my testicles dragging a log through three feet of snow in a Russian winter.

> **Assistant:** So, any questions?

Goddammit, I need to stop daydreaming.

> **Me:** …

> **Assistant:** I need to repeat myself again, don't I?

> **Me:** I am so, so sorry.

I was able to stop thinking about my testicles in training long enough to hear her tell me that I will need at least two full days of rest. During this rest period, I will be able to take a prescription of painkillers they'll give me because I'll be sore.

I can only imagine how sore I will be. I used to be a catcher in little league, and one time I got hit in the nads with a ball so hard that I threw up all over Mary Jane Wingleton's couch in her basement. Wait. Hold on. I'm confusing baseball with a party I went to when I was 15. Never mind.

Stay in school, kids.

Nevertheless, two days of rest while sitting in bed or on the couch and a bottle of Vicodin sounds like a pretty sweet deal, right? The only way I could imagine this scenario getting any better was if she told me I could only eat hot dogs during recovery. I mean, aside from someone digging into my squishy parts with a scalpel, the aftermath was sounding decent.

I asked her how many pills were in the prescription. She said she wasn't sure so I asked if I could maybe get one ball done at a time so I could stretch the painkillers out a bit, but she seemed to be a little agitated with me at that point so I didn't really push the issue.

She also told me that I would need to keep ice on my crotch for two days and do no heavy lifting for two weeks. The "no heavy lifting" thing is easy for me because I don't even like hoisting myself off the toilet. If they made toilets like those chairs old people buy that stand them up so they could just walk off, I would probably poop more. The ice thing sounds a little harsh, though. However, all this is needed because there is a chance my testicles can balloon to the size of grapefruits if I don't try to keep the swelling down.

That's right: BALLS THE SIZE OF GRAPEFRUITS.

Although grapefruit balls may be a normal look for the guy who models the giant penis pictures in the urologist's office, this would not be good for me, a man just over five feet tall. I will try very hard to avoid grapefruit balls – as not only will they be extremely large on my little frame, but also they will probably throw off my center of gravity, like having six bricks stuffed in a fanny pack. Also, grapefruit balls are something you certainly won't want to pop in your mouth after just brushing your teeth.

Okay. So to recap, I have ice, pills, and lots of rest.

I have to say, this post-op period was sounding sweet.

That is when she gave me a job to do. This is also the part where I got really, really confused.

> **Assistant:** To make sure the procedure worked, you will
> need to ejaculate 25 times.

She told me that I would have to ejaculate (the clinical term is "whack off") 25 times after the operation. Then I would need to come back to the office and bring in the 26th sample with me, so they could test it in the lab to see if all my little swimmers had vacated the pool.

Wait a minute.

What do I have to do? I THOUGHT I WAS DONE WITH ALL THAT EJACULATING NONSENSE.

I always thought of it this way:

Let's say there is a tunnel. The tunnel leads to a baby factory. Cars come into this tunnel all the time and exit the other side at various speeds and/or frequency based on the amount of porn that the owner of the tunnel watches. When the cars exit the tunnel they arrive at the baby factory and if one lucky car is chosen as "Employee of the Month," he gets to make a baby.

Now let's pretend a construction crew closes the road just before the entrance to the tunnel.

If no cars can get into the tunnel, then no cars can exit the tunnel. If no cars can exit the tunnel, then no one can get to the baby factory to be named the "star worker" and no babies can be made. This sounds like it should be made into a sequel for the *Cars* movie franchise but rated NC-17. I hope they don't get Owen Wilson to voice this.

The doctor's assistant, though, seemed to be telling me that cars *are* exiting the tunnel. FROM WHERE? Is there a hidden onramp inside the tunnel somewhere?

I was beyond lost trying to wrap my head around this. The car analogy was not helping.

I have to admit, as much as I am an eager student when it comes to working my own anatomy, I have no real idea how anything of reproductive importance actually functions.

The penis goes up.

The penis goes down.

Sometimes the penis does not go up no matter how much you try to talk him into it. Sometimes the penis looks good dressed in a Barbie outfit with a face drawn on it and likes to be called Madame Consuela.

That is all I know.

When someone tells you that the carpool that drops your swimmers off at the pool is going to be shut down and they have no other ride, I had to wonder: *who is jumping off the diving board?*

So I raised my hand.

> **Assistant:** Um. You have a question? You don't have to raise-

> **Me:** Ejaculate? What the hell am I ejaculating?

> **Assistant:** Well, what do you THINK comes out?

> **Me:** I just thought it went like this:

I took a small breath and puffed out a little air.

Foof

Really, I had no idea. I thought that once this procedure was all said and done, the only thing that would come out of the little guy would be a tiny poof of air. If there was a woman down there maybe her hair would flip up for a second (like when you are hot and try to blow on your own forehead) kind of like she was getting hit by a miniature hair dryer.

Foof

There was complete and utter silence for a few seconds. I think she was a little taken aback by the fact that I puffed on her face to simulate the effect I was going for. I find many times that audience participation is key to getting your point across. In this instance, though, I think she was maybe three seconds away from calling security before she realized I was dead serious.

She then began to clarify.

> **Assistant** [fixing the hair I had blown back from her forehead]: Um. No. It's something called "seminal fluid."

> **Me:** I am going to shoot out Florida State College students?

Assistant: Those are the Seminoles.

Me: Oh. Good. That sounded painful.

Then I held my hand up for a high-five but at that point I don't think she was in the mood. She continued to explain that this whole little cocktail *(please note here that she actually used that term so I cannot be held responsible for my giggling)* that comes out of there. Sperm is only 1% of the mix, while the rest is stuff bubbled up from your nether regions in an area a little higher than where they make the snip. THAT stuff coming from the area closer to the tunnel exit is called "seminal fluid."

Me: Ah. So why did they name it after Florida State?

Assistant: I would like you to leave now.

I got dressed and left, but not before making my appointment for the procedure. Let the countdown begin.

I go back in ten days for it.

I could really use that Vicodin prescription right now.

Chapter 3

Prep Work

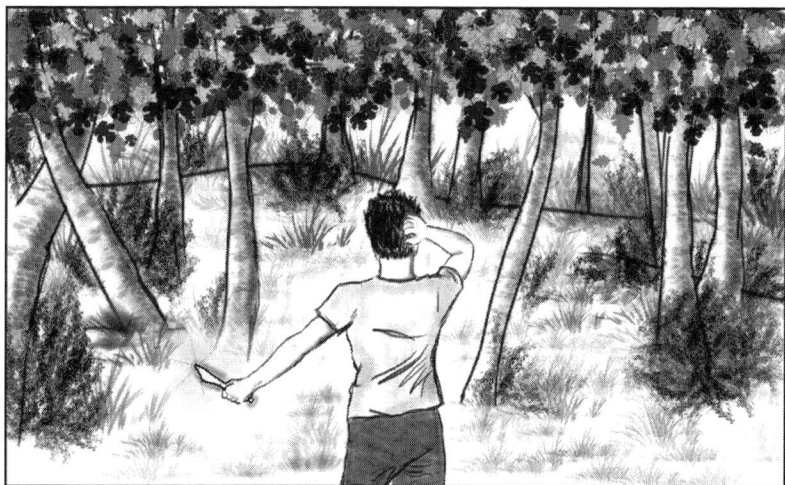

Why isn't "manscaping" a real word in spell-checker? Now my resume has all these red squiggly lines on it.

Day 11

Hi, Diary.

I'm sorry that I have been a bit absent as of late. Most of my time has been spent chasing my kids all around because children cannot simply stand still for more than three seconds without the use of Benadryl or some other magic serum.

It is exhausting.

Also exhausting is finding out your seven-year-old had unsuccessfully tried to forge her mother's signature on a note that she was supposed to bring home and have us sign. The note explained that my daughter had been caught at school taking pencils out of someone's desk. To acknowledge this, a note was sent home.

It was returned to the teacher signed, alright, but not by either one of us. My daughter had used a pencil to forge my wife's name, which was also spelled incorrectly with one of the letters written backward. This is why some animals eat their young.

On the flipside, I had to be a chaperone on my son's first field trip. This was actually fun because we got to ride in a bus and I was the only father amidst all the mommy chaperones. Had the kids not actually been on the bus, I am assuming I would be writing here about some crazed sex party or something. However, since kids ruin everything, all I have is a story that goes, "We went to an apple orchard. There were apples. The end."

In addition, I still have not shaved my "area."

I have been working up the courage to do it. I've known my groin for many, many years and it has always looked the same. I don't know that I am ready to change all that yet, but I know I will have to do it very soon. It's going to be weird to look down there and see stuff I don't recognize anymore. It is probably like coming home to discover that all your furniture has been rearranged while you were gone and, oh yeah, someone also removed all the carpeting.

I am going to miss my carpeting.

Although, I think I might be able to find my beanbag chairs in my body's rumpus room a little easier.

Day 13

8:00 AM

No real updates but I figured today I would start researching how to shave myself. I plan on going out to the library after work and see what I can find. I hope that they have picture books.

2:00 PM

Went to the library during a work break and asked if they had picture books showing men shaving the male anatomy.

Related: I have been banned from the library.

Off to the bookstores.

3:30 PM

I am no longer welcome in the local Barnes & Noble and also Jim the manager there is kind of an asshole.

I guess I'll try Google.

9:45 PM

1,499,000.

That is how many results come up in a Google search for "How to shave your balls."

1.5 MILLION ARTICLES.

1.5 million posts on manscaping were returned, and these are just the sites in ENGLISH. I am sure that if I expanded my search criteria, I would be able to find out how to shave my nuts on an even greater, international scale. Maybe I'd learn how to trim my crotch to look like Disney World shrubbery or a tiny version of the Eiffel Tower or even the Egyptian pyramids.

The number of results astounds me. I am finding it hard to believe that in an area roughly the size of a drink coaster you can have 1.5 million options on how to trim your hedges. Hey, Internet, I don't want to pursue a career in cosmetology, I just need to shave my nuts.

I may just go out on a limb and try this on my own. I once had a Chia Pet so, really, how tough could this be? Then again, my Chia Pet was not attached to my groin and did not bleed. Maybe I should practice on a bonsai tree first. Come to think of it, I have no idea how to trim a bonsai tree, either. Nor do I have an elderly Asian man in the area who can take me under his wing and train me on how to do so. I already know karate so I'd only need the old Asian man for his bonsai-trimming skills but, nope, not a one.

I'm starting to think that New Hampshire sucks as far as diversity goes.

Day 14

Today was a day of reflection for me.

Actually, only half the day was for reflection. I spent the first half of the day watching a Karate Kid marathon. I originally started it because I wanted to see how Mr. Miagi trimmed his bonsai tree, but then I was hooked and time got away from me. Suffice it to say I am now 6 hours older and no better at karate or trimming bonsai trees, but I still think Elisabeth Shue is crazy hot.

With the distractions of bonsais and sexy Shues out of the way, my thoughts turned to the weight of my decision. Specifically, not having more kids without needing a vasectomy reversal. I concluded that I am *never* having more children because to hell with the idea of someone going back down there to hack me up again. Vasectomy once, shame on me. Vasectomy twice, I have issues and would probably enjoy BDSM.

Nevertheless, it got me thinking about all the cool parts of being a dad. I know someday my kids are going to be older and my son will someday be able to wipe his own ass (thank God because the kid craps like he eats planets), and maybe I will miss the times when they were babies or little and needed me to hold their hands and help them do everything. As much as raising kids is hard and can really suck sometimes, there are other times when it is really really good.

First, there was that time that my two-year-old daughter, just potty training, realized that the poop nuggets she just left in her potty-training toilet could be made into a smiley face if she reached in and rearranged them by hand. It was both hysterical and gross at the same time. It was also a realization that we probably shouldn't leave a toddler alone in a room with her own poop.

There were her dance recitals, where we would spend the first ten minutes of each recital taking pictures, laughing at the small children trying to move in perfect unison and failing miserably. Then we would spend the next three hours watching the older kids who we honestly didn't care about, but now everyone's stuck watching teenagers dance and yelling things like "BOOOOORING" and "BRING BACK THE FUNNY LITTLE KIDS" and sometimes being escorted out by security.

There was that time we took the kids to Sea World in Florida and were looking at the shark tank. It wasn't Great Whites or anything like that – just sand sharks and stingrays – but you could buy these gross little packs of dead squid to feed them. We were all standing by the edge of the shark tank, grabbing dead squid and throwing them into the aquarium, when it came to my son's turn. Cam took the squid and heaved it with all the energy his little body could muster. As his tiny hand came forward, he hooked the inside of my eyeglasses with his finger and proceeded to launch them off my face and ten feet into the shark pool.

PLOOP

I watched, horrified and with extremely blurred vision now, as my glasses sunk three feet to the bottom of the shark pool. I was stunned. I could not reach them and – no Great Whites or not – there was zero chance I was wading into a pool of sharks to go get my glasses. I would much rather be blind than eaten alive at Sea World. It was then, at that very moment, a stingray sauntered over and placed himself right on top of them in an apparent effort to try to eat them.

OH NO.

Thankfully, stingrays apparently have no stomach for corrective lenses and a Sea World employee was able to fish them out for me. Yes, that pun was intentional, and no, this is not an apology for it.

I know that as my kids get older the experiences are going to get better. I will be able to have intelligent conversations with them that go beyond who their favorite person on *The Wiggles* is. I just wonder if I am going to miss them when they are this little, enough to want another one.

Then again, I am almost 40.

Screw that.

Day 16

I shaved my balls today.

[trumpets blare]

Yep. It's done.

Down there, right now at this very moment, is as smoooooooth as a baby's bum. Actually, that is probably the worst analogy I could have possibly made.

I work with a woman named Kristin whose husband manscapes. I know this because she is essentially my work-wife and we discuss pretty much everything. Personally, I hate knowing the exact dates of her menstrual cycle or about that time she shit in her friend's car or her husband's preference for dressing up like a chicken in the bedroom, but it's better than watching my boss give PowerPoint Presentations so I just listen to her and then later try to forget the nightmarish things.

Of course, Kristin knows everything that is going on in regards to this vasectomy, so when I told her that I needed to crop my winky whiskers she got all excited. I'm not sure why, exactly. We have never had sex or anything but, hey, if she is excited about me shaving my junk I am not going to rain on her parade. When a woman seems excited about your crotch you roll with it. I was raised to be a gentleman.

As soon as I told her, she started saying stuff like, "Jeff shaves and it is so nice. His balls are like butter."

This immediately got me thinking "butter balls" which got me to thinking about turkeys. Now every time I see Jeff at social gatherings all I can picture is a shaved turkey in his pants. I really need to stop talking to Kristin, now that I am writing all this stuff down.

So let's not say "smooth as a baby's bum." I'm going to say "smooth like butter."

My balls are smooth like butter.

I am not sure why I've never done this sooner. I grew up during a time where men were men and the bigger your bush, the more land you could claim rightfully as your own. Because of this, men just let things grow wild down there and even sometimes shampooed using Miracle-Gro just to claim bragging rights over the next guy's chub-shrub. We are living in modern times now, though, and having a massive pubic-hair farm just so you can own more land also means having to do more yard work and, honestly, who needs that shit. Yard work is so tiring.

I guess the main reason I never trimmed my man-garden was mainly out of fear. Things are BUMPY down there. I have cut my face enough times while shaving to know that running a razor blade across something the consistency of half-filled water balloons with the texture of old corduroy probably will not end well.

As I was going through those 1.5 million "how-to" articles, I found a common thread: most women apparently *like* this look. I know my friend Kristin likes it, but she also likes her husband dressing like a chicken during sex so I typically discount all of her recommendations. This, though, this was information from THE INTERNET so it had to be true.

I find all this a little hard to believe, though, because I once shaved my chest. I am not a super-hairy guy but hairy enough to catch crackers when I'm eating. I know that sounds gross but it has saved me a lot of time cleaning crackers up off the floor and also I get to eat them because food in your own chest hair does not require a five-second rule. Essentially, having chest hair has probably saved me ones of dollars in food costs over the years. I should probably pass this information on to the Feed the Children program.

I forget where I was going with all of this.

OH. Yes. Ladies digging this look.

After I shaved my chest, I walked downstairs, shirtless. My wife was on the phone at the time.

> **Me** [leaning against the wall]: Heyyyyyyyyyy.

> **Wife** [turning, with the phone to her ear]: OHMYGOD WHAT DID YOU DO YOU LOOK LIKE A HAIRLESS MOLE.

> **Me:** Thanks. Tell whoever is on the phone I said "hi."

I only hoped she would not be on the phone when I showed her the results of what I was about to do. If she was, I hoped it wasn't with her mom again, at least.

Speaking of hairless moles, let me get back to the story of shaving my groin.

The first step in doing this was to find an acceptable razor. I obviously could not use the same razor that I use for my face because that would be like transferring my face germs onto my own crotch. I would never be able to use that razor to shave my face again because ew. Someone else's face germs on my crotch? Sure. My own face on my crotch? No, thank you. I like myself, but not that much.

My other option was to just use my face razor and then throw it out and grow a beard. However, my beard only comes out in patches and clumps, and whenever I try to grow one people think I've contracted a disease. This is great at work because it allows me to avoid people, but looking like I've stuck balls of lint to random sections of my face is not great for one's social life. Given all of this, it was essential that I find a new razor to use.

This became a problem.

Razors these days are not like they used to be. When I was a kid, we had disposable Bic Razors with a single blade. Light, simple, and easy to use, there was no place these razors couldn't go except maybe out of the country because razors cannot carry a passport.

Nowadays, though, all razors have fourteen blades, three lubricating strips, fancy LED lighting and a cash bar. THEY ARE HUGE. This is where I have a major issue when it comes to manscaping.

I am small – five feet, three inches tall and a size seven shoe. I should mention those measurements were taken on a warm day while people were holding onto my neck and ankles and yanking in opposite directions. I am certainly not setting any records in the length and girth departments as far as Li'l Willy and his two amigos go, by any means. With the size of shaving instruments these days, it was going to be like rolling a sheet of plywood over a pencil.

So the smallest razor I could find was a Mach 3. The Mach 3 comes with three blades but, contrary to its name, cannot fly on its own, as I discovered while throwing it in the aisle at Target. It was still huge, though, compared to my old one-bladed Bic Razor from 1983. On the bright side, I figured that with a razor this big, this whole process should be over quickly. On the not so bright side, I did not think I had room on my penis to actually move this thing back an entire stroke.

I got undressed, hopped in the shower and while holding the razor in one hand I looked down to see what I had to deal with.

It was a jungle down there.

Honestly, I don't think I had ever taken a really good look at my junk. Of course, I knew what was down there and how to handle it, given my decades of manual practice, but I'd never taken a hard look at it. I felt like I was discovering a Mayan ruin. An unshaved male crotch is basically a square-foot of thick underbrush, with a couple of grassy knolls off to the south and a temple rising from the north. After careful consideration, I now believe that JFK's shooter was not on a grassy knoll in Dallas, but rather hiding out in someone's unshaved testicular region.

How was I supposed to navigate all of this with just this stupid razor? I felt like a lumberjack approaching a dense forest that needed to be cleared but all I brought with me was a butter knife.

I could not, in good conscience, just start shaving this mess.

Then, I had a brainstorm:

MY BEARD TRIMMER.

I mentally added it to my list of things that would need to be thrown out after doing this, and then hopped out of the shower. I grabbed my trimmer and moved this tree-trimming party over to the toilet.

Pants down, squatting over my toilet, I start hacking away.

We have all seen the videos of soldiers having their heads shaved when they join the military. The whole process for them takes about ten seconds and three swipes of the trimmer. I can tell you that, after 15 minutes of navigating my crotch using various angles of attack and dislocating both of my shoulders, clearing a massive ball-bush is much harder.

How my trimmer did not get jammed, I have no idea. There were a few minutes where it sounded like it wanted to give up — and I would not have blamed it — but it kept chugging along like The Little Trimmer that Could.

Lil Trimmer that Could: I THINK I CAN TRIM PUBES I THINK I CAN TRIM PUBES

Kids on other Side of Mountain: Why would you bring us all of this?!?!

Eventually, I felt I had my pasture whittled down enough where I could take care of the rest with the razor. I stood up from the toilet ready to head into the shower to finish the party, but not before taking one glance back to see what I had done.

It looked like there was a brown guinea pig floating in the toilet.

It also looked like someone emptied the vacuum cleaner bag of a hair salon all over that area of the bathroom. Not everything had fallen straight down where I had intended, and the toilet was covered and surrounded by approximately 15,000 stray hairs that had apparently taken flight on the wind like a new batch of baby spiders.

I did what any respectful husband would do. I took a tissue and whisked them all into the heating duct. I figured I would wait until my wife was in the bathroom, then crank the heat on, and listen to her scream.

Then I started the hot water and stepped into the shower, ready to finish the job. This is where it got tricky.

Using a trimmer is one thing. You can hack back and forth with wild abandon.

Being super-careful is not required with a trimmer. It is pretty much like painting the wall in a room. You can just slop paint all over the place willy-nilly, but when you get down to the details you need to use a little finesse.

Standing there, razor in hand, I was a bit nervous.

What was I thinking? Tearing my hair out to have a doctor tear my vas deferens out. IT SOUNDED LIKE INSANITY.

However, it was already too late. I was in too deep with the consultation and the appointment and now I had already partially manscaped my way to a look of genital mange. I had no choice but to press on.

It was do-or-die time and I was now faced with a myriad of choices:

1. With the grain or against the grain?

2. Side to side? Up or down?

3. I could go for a Snickers bar. I'm hungry. I think I've been in here for three hours.

4. Just shave the berries?

5. Just shave the twig?

6. Shave the twig and maybe just *one* berry? Like Jekyll and Hyde testicles.

7. Is "the Hitler" look acceptable for your genitals? Or is it considered a faux pas even down there?

I decided to go full-Kojak. Lex Luthor. Yul Brynner in *The King and I*. That kid in the *Avatar* cartoon and maybe I could just keep a little arrow design for effect. Nah.

Bald.

I took the razor in my shaky little hand and started shaving. This is actually more exhausting than I imagined it would be because shaving things with bumps, curves, and irregular angles with a butthole sitting right next-door means you have to try to make things *flat*. I'm not huge on cardio, so the dexterity required to take a single round bumpy testicle and flatten it out using one hand, while simultaneously trying to shave the hair off it with the other, should probably be an obstacle on *American Ninja Warrior.*

> **Announcer:** Well he really flew through the rope ladder and salmon ladder challenges, but now he's onto the testicle-shaving portion of the course and OH NO HE LET GO TOO EARLY. What a tragedy. Oh, looks like he is going back to get the nut he just lopped off.

It is terrifying.

So I pulled on them. I pulled and I pulled as if I was trying to make a bed in the army and bounce a quarter off it when I was done. I had no desire to hack my balls off by leaving them all limp and lumpy so, instead, I grabbed them firmly in one hand, stretched them upwards to within an inch of my chin and shaved.

I had no idea the scrotum was so flexible. I will never ever look at a Stretch Armstrong doll the same way again.

Carefully, I moved on. Stretching. Twisting. Bending. I pulled to the left. I pulled to the right. I pulled straight up. I did the Hokey Pokey. Over the river and through the woods until, finally, the job was done.

Tired and hungry, at looked at my masterpiece.

It looked bigger.

Seriously.

Now, I know that everything is relative but my little toy soldier looked like he put on a few pounds. Imagine if the Washington Monument only had its top half exposed because the bottom half was buried in afro wigs. Then someone takes all the wigs away and you are, like, "Wow, it looks taller than I thought." That was me just then:

standing in the shower thinking my Washington Monument looked much more impressive without the bottom half buried in a thicket of afros.

Why did it have a tan line?

I could not figure that part out. The far end of him was darker than the part that used to be all covered up, with a distinctive demarcation line showing exactly where my hair used to be. It was as if George Hamilton took his clothes off to reveal that he had milky white legs. Also, I am now nicknaming my penis "George Hamilton." I've just decided.

Nevertheless, I survived the ordeal. I am shaved for the procedure. I did not cut anything off. I had all my parts and could see them now, clear as day.

I feel like a kid with a new toy.

Talk to you later, Diary. I'm off to play with it.

Day 17

[singing]: Tomorrow, tomorrow. I don't love you, tomorrow. I wish you were further than a day awayyyyyyy...

I am nervous for tomorrow.

It's Thursday, and I have taken today and tomorrow off to give me the entire weekend to recover. The folks at work had a little going away party for my sperm and it was equally touching and disturbing. If there is one thing I am thankful for, it is the support of my friends. If there is a second thing I am thankful for, it's that our Human Resources Department isn't strict because I am almost positive a "sperm going away party" complete with semen-shaped balloons violates some part of our harassment code.

On a side note, I told Kristin she was right about the whole "shaved" thing.

EVERYTHING IS SMOOTH LIKE BUTTER.

I mean, not to the point I would spread them out on toast, but whatever.

Now I am wondering what else Kristin and her husband might be right about. Maybe I should look into this "dressing like a chicken" thing.

Day 18: D-Day is V-Day

Today is the day.

"Vasectomy Day," to be exact. I checked the Internet and there is no "National Celebrate Your Vasectomy Day" which makes sense because the parade would just be a bunch of guys limping along while holding bags of frozen peas on their crotch.

Slowest. Parade. Ever.

In approximately four hours, my twins will be exposed, examined and prodded by people who make way more money than I do, much like Liam Neeson's daughter in *Taken.* This would be a great time for Liam Neeson to show off his special set of skills and come rescue my testicles from certain mutilation.

They will call it *Taken 4: The Final Cut* and my scrotum will be played by Steve Buscemi.

In preparation for Vasectomy Day, I have done the following:

1) Showered

2) Shaved my downstairs again because I don't want a 5 o'clock shadow like I have a couple of little George Clooney doppelgangers down there

3) Applied Britney Spears' new perfume to said doppelgangers to make this a pleasurable experience for the doctor

4) Bought a jockstrap

I have not worn a jockstrap since Little League, back when I was a 200-pound eight-year-old who managed one accidental hit in his entire three-year career. I remember the hit fondly because it turned out to be an accidental GRAND SLAM. How a kid with the same gravitational mass as Pluto managed to not only hit a ball but also get all the way around four bases is a testament to how bad the opposing team was.

My poor mother, so surprised that I actually hit the ball and was doing cardio for the first time in my life without the aid of a Twinkie dangling from a string in front of my face, leaped from her chair in excitement. Unfortunately, she was at the top of a small hill and tripped when she jumped up, causing herself to fall and subsequently roll all the way to the bottom while yelling:

"YaaayyyyyyyyyyyOWyayyOWWyayaOOOFyayyyyy."

On a side note, it's really hard to concentrate on circling the bases when out of the corner of your eye you can see your mother tumbling down an embankment.

The doctor's office called me yesterday to remind me of my appointment. Yeah. Thank you for the reminder, Doc. I had completely forgotten that I was scheduled to undergo life-changing ball surgery that has kept me up with anxiety attacks for the past week. I was going to get fondue at that same time, so it's a good thing you called. Jerks.

They told me I would need a ride home and should also bring a jockstrap. I thought the ride home was a no-brainer because I assumed I'd be in traction or have a couple of tiny casts or something that would make driving difficult. The jockstrap is apparently to "keep everything together," according to the woman who called me. She obviously has not seen me because most of my stuff down there has been together since birth and they really hate being separated. One time my penis left for a walkabout in Australia and man, my balls were pretty blue.

I am putting a sticky-note on this page to remind myself to come back and take out all the really bad puns. I'm not sure if that one is going to make the cut.

Or the one in that last sentence, either.

Maybe I'll just put two sticky-notes here to be safe.

I took my son to the local Walmart in search of a jockstrap. If I was going to buy one, there was certainly no way I was going to pay a ridiculous price for it at a sporting goods store, and plus I also needed deodorant and beef jerky.

Walking around the sporting goods section of Walmart took a lot longer than we expected because Cam and I spent 20 extra minutes playing with the fishing rods, pretending to catch people walking by the aisles. Cam wasn't picky about who he'd pretend to reel in, but I was focused on not casting my line towards any of the big men in camouflage heading towards the gun section.

I never did actually see anything called a "jockstrap." The closest thing I found said, "Full Supporter with Cup" on the package. Inside was an elastic thing that looked like it would make a good slingshot and the "cup" which looked like something Jason Voorhees would wear as an oxygen mask.

Then I remembered what the woman on the phone said.

"Buy two jockstraps because there will be seepage."

She was lovely.

I have a 32-inch waist. This meant I had to choose between the one for a 28-to-32-inch waist and one for a 32-to-36-inch waist. The cup size was much bigger for the larger supporter, so I went with the smaller one because I did not want everything to be all flippity-floppity in there like kids in a bouncy house. In addition, I would only need this for a little while and my son could use it for when he got older and played sports.

Son: Dad, I want to play baseball.

Me: Well, son. I have something for you that I've been saving for a while until you were old enough to need it.

Son: [opens mahogany case with phenomenal interior lighting that illuminates our family jockstrap inside]

Me: It was mine back when-

Son: Never mind. I'll just play Xbox.

We started leaving Walmart with jockstraps in hand. I fancy myself a good dad and since it is important to let your child participate in things to feel involved, I let him carry the supporters through the store. He was excited to carry them because I told him they were slingshots.

We stood in the checkout line and Cam immediately decided that this would be a great time to see if he could juggle.

He could not juggle.

Both containers hit the linoleum floor and burst open, sending the contents scattering past the line of people standing behind us.

Son: OH NO DAD, OUR SLINGSHOTS!

I found myself hunting along the ground, searching for two cups through a crowd of Walmart shoppers, none of whom would pick them up for me. Honestly, I could not blame them. This was Walmart and they were probably used and returned anyway.

I finally found them, haphazardly stuck them back into the packages and checked out.

When we got home, I went up to my bedroom and tried one on.

SONOFABITCH.

I should have gone with the bigger size.

I looked like a watermelon being stuffed into a sausage casing. Apparently, the 28-to-32-inch waistband is made for 28 inches but maxes out at 32 inches. It felt and looked like I had somehow managed to put on a toddler's bathing suit.

The entire contents of my crotch were somehow shoehorned into the cup, with some parts here and there peeking out around the corners. It was like a clown car for genitals.

Wife: How does it fit?

Me: [passes out]

I ended up running back out to a sporting goods store and got actual "jockstraps." These are essentially thongs with a cloth tent area for keeping my package all together. They also look like they would make better slingshots, so I am very happy with the purchase.

That's it. I am all packed and ready to go.

I'm going to guess I am not going to be in the mood to be sitting around typing in a diary later, so I will check in tomorrow. If there is nothing on the next pages and this turns out to be my last entry, that means I died on the operating room table with my genitals fully exposed to the elements and that my kids are probably reading this right now.

Kids: I love you. Grow up to be kind and loving. I will always be with you and will always be proud.

Also, don't ever look in the bottom drawer of daddy's nightstand. You may never recover.

Chapter 4

Go Time

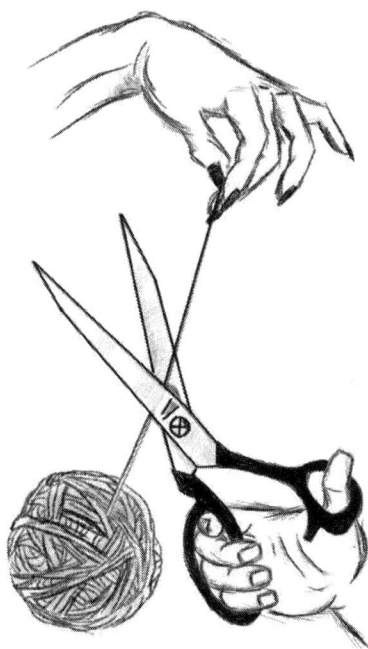

Entrepreneurial Idea #812:

A vasectomy clinic near the exit of Disney World.

Pins and Needles

It's over.

At approximately 11:30 AM yesterday, the fat lady sang her songs for me and my two little bouncing boys.

Her first song was a lovely rendition of AC/DC's "Big Balls" done acapella-style, followed by "You Don't Know What You've Got Til It's Gone" and then, for some reason, "99 Luftballons." Why did the woman only have 99 luftballons? Couldn't she have sprung for one more luftballon to make it an even 100 luftballons? These things keep me up at night.

I am taking Vicodin right now.

I am writing to you, dear Diary, from the couch with a giant bag of ice on my lap. The constant haziness that the drugs are inducing is helping to take my mind off the sheer horror I witnessed just a scant 24 hours ago.

I will do my best to give a full rundown, but please note that there may be random bouts of puking interspersed between the words as I attempt to retell it, so this may take some effort.

I arrived at the urologist's office carrying a duffle bag that included a change of underwear and one of the jockstraps that Cam and I bought. When we left the house, Cam was using the cup portion as a Darth Vader mask and slinging Matchbox cars across the room with the elastic part. I did not have the heart to tell him what he was actually wearing, and it was cute to hear him doing the breathing through it.

I was in jogging pants because I was told to wear loose clothing. I was also wearing my grandmother's housecoat with pictures of fruit baskets on it. Turns out I only needed to wear loose pants, but I may keep this mumu dress on anyway because it is actually quite liberating and the fabric doesn't chafe my nipples.

My wife could not stop smiling the entire time, all the way from the moment we woke up until the second they called me into the room. It is always a bit disconcerting when someone takes a sincere pleasure in your mutilation, but women have been playing the "labor pains" card since the days of the caveman so I was looking forward to getting a little bit of payback.

Woman: I birthed humans from this tiny orifice!

Man: Well, I had my testicles cut open!

Woman: I birthed humans and also have a menstrual cyc-

Man: OKAY YOU WIN JUST STOP TALKING ABOUT THAT LALALALA I CAN'T HEAR YOU.

The office door opened and a nice woman in scrubs poked her head out and said, "Rodney?"

I held the SO YOU HAVE AN STD, NOW WHAT? pamphlet that I was reading a little higher to cover my face, but my wife nudged me off the chair. Okay, lady. I get it. Childbirth. Jesus, let it go.

I got up and followed the woman into the room. As the door closed I turned to give a final glimpse back at my wife, but she was already gone to get an iced coffee. I hoped she would get two or three because it would probably feel good to have an iced hazelnut propped between my legs on the way home. I could still hear her laughing as her car exited the parking lot and down the street.

The nurse ushered me into the same room where I had my original consultation. She told me to remove my pants, put on a hospital johnnie, hop up on the table, and wait for the doctor.

Me: Can I keep my mumu on?

The nurse just looked back, and without saying a word, closed the door behind her. I guess that meant "yes."

I sat there in the office, alone and violently dry-heaving, for only a few minutes before the door on the opposite side of the room opened and a man walked in. As he introduced himself as "Doctor Cannotrememberhisname," the door opened again, and a ridiculously attractive nurse came in. Like, she was silly pretty as in, *normally I would have to pay someone like that a few hundred bucks to even consider looking at my junk* silly pretty.

Fantastic. I was starting to get the feeling that the person in charge of doing the hiring here previously managed a Hooters franchise.

Then, just when I thought it could not get any more awkward, it did.

Doctor: Okay, lie back, please. Let's see what we're
dealing with here.

I laid down on that stupid sterile paper and looked down. Hottie McHotnurse was stationed on the left side of the table and the doctor was on the right. It looked like they were about to play a game of checkers.

Me: KING ME!

Doctor: Excuse me?

Me: It looks like you're going to play checkers down there
you know what, never mind, just do your thing. I'll be
up here just entertaining myself.

He raised up my johnnie.

>**Me:** TADAAA!

>**Doctor:** Please stop.

Then, staring intensely at my goolies, he said it:

>**Doctor:** Wow. Hey, nice job down there.

>**Me:** Um. What?

>**Doctor:** Great job trimming up.

Awesome. The doctor just complimented me on my mad ball-shaving skillz.

I mean, here is a guy who probably sees, like, 20 patients a day. That's 40 balls a day. That is roughly 9,800 balls this man sees annually if you factor in the three weeks of vacation he gets. I do not know if he sees balls on vacation, but if he does, we are talking about a man looking at 10,000 testicles per annum. That is Pamela Anderson territory.

All those nuts and he complimented MINE.

I blushed.

I was suddenly feeling good about myself. Thoughts of accepting some sort of "Manscaping of the Year" award floated through my head.

That would be a weird parade.

Then all that joy quickly changed as soon as the needle emerged.

OH NO.

Needles.

I hate needles.

I hate needles almost as much as I hate spiders. Actually, that needle was about to go straight into one of my nuts, so there was about to be some major jockeying for the top spot on my "Things I Hate" list. The only way this could be worse was if the needle was full of spiders OH MY GOD WHY DOES MY BRAIN DO THIS TO ME.

Doctor: This is going to hurt.

Wow. Way to sugarcoat it, Doc.

But he wasn't kidding.

I pinched my fingers and bit my lip as hard as I could. It did not help. I could feel him grabbing Mr. Lefty in one hand and then kind of spreading him out as if he was trying to turn it into a picnic blanket. I looked down to see what he was doing just in time to watch the needle go in.

It burned like a thousand suns.

If Hell is an actual real place and you are doomed to spend your own eternal torment repeating the worst moment of your life, then getting a needle in my sack is certainly one of the top contenders. I think even Jack Bauer from *24* would consider this cruel and unusual punishment for trying to get information out of a terrorist.

Instinctively, my right knee shot up and I almost took the doctor's skull off.

Doctor: Easy, buddy. Relax.

Okay. I'll relax. I'll relax as soon as you are done puncturing my scrotum with hypodermic needles, you sociopath. I could only assume the syringes contained sulfuric acid *seriously why was this burning so much.*

Doctor: Okay. One down. Two to go.

Two? Two to go? I only have two balls, so why was I getting three shots? Did they find an extra nut hiding out down there somewhere? I didn't under-

The shot to my right testicle went in and felt ten times worse than the left one. My right knee shot upwards again, nearly decapitating the doctor. He was starting to get pissed but I could not think of any other way he could punish me that would be worse than what he was currently doing so I might as well try to kill him.

Two shots down, one to go.

Honestly, I don't even know where the third one went in. I was just concentrating on trying to keep my legs down and hoping my whimpering was at a low enough volume that the hot nurse could not hear it.

Doctor: Okay. Done. Let's get started.

Done?

Started?

Those two words together did not make sense. Then I realized he was saying that he was done piercing my gonads with tiny spears. Whatever he shot into me with the first two must have worked because I didn't feel the third needle go in. That was good, because if I had felt it I would probably be typing this from prison while facing assault charges.

Injections done, it was time to move onto the task at hand.

That is right about the time I needed a bucket.

Puff, My Magic Dragon

Doctor: OHMYGOD ARE YOU GOING TO THROW UP?

I violently nodded my head "YES" because either I was having a reaction to the Novocain or the sight of the nurse wheeling over the instrument table hit home a little too hard. Whatever it was, I could feel the blood rushing out of my face, about to spray the two Pop Tarts I had for breakfast all over the doctor.

The nurse quickly handed me one of those plastic things that you would pee into while in a hospital bed. That curved, shallow thing that looks like a kidney but is better suited for holding in front of your mouth so you can make yourself look like you have a big smile or are really sad and frowny. I made it into a frown because that was how I was feel-

Nurse: STOP MAKING FACES WITH IT, IT'S TO THROW UP INTO.

Me: Oh. I'm good. You would have been safe, anyway. I always only throw up on people who are about to make an incision in my testicles, just for future reference.

Then I turned that pee-cup frown upside-down and made it into a smile.

I handed her back the little dish and laid back down. I could hear the doctor rummaging around with some instruments as they both wheeled themselves closer to my junk. I had not had anyone's face this close to my pelvis since well before my second child was born.

I could feel a tiny bit of tugging down there. The closest analogy I can come up with is that it felt like getting a nibble on the line when you are fishing, and the fishing pole moves a little. I haven't been fishing since the last time I went with my dad when I was, like, eight years old and he hooked my ear while casting his line. I screamed and I screamed but he kept on trying to cast the line thinking it was stuck on a tree branch but, nope, he had pierced his son's ear and was desperately trying to yank me into the pond. This is probably why I don't like to eat fish or won't go fishing or talk to my dad.

The feeling was a bit disconnected. I knew something was happening because I could feel him yanking on things but it didn't hurt at all. I stared straight up at the ceiling because I feared that if I *did* look down I would actually throw up and it would get all inside my balls. The resulting infection would probably start the zombie apocalypse. I have already been a "patient zero" once and am not eager to do that again. That story is for an entirely different diary.

Then a conversation between the doctor and nurse started. I wasn't a fan of this because, personally, I am terrible at multitasking. I can barely think and speak at the same time, so I couldn't imagine performing testicle surgery while discussing my grandmother's <u>favorite</u> no-bake Swedish meatball recipe. Yet, here they were chit-chatting like teenagers in a movie theater.

Nurse: Remember that guy that came in here last week?

Doctor: The 22-year old?

Nurse: Mmmmm. Yeah. Now HE was nice looking.

Seriously? What in the sweet hell was going on? My cleanly shaven marbles were numbed up, eviscerated and spread out all over who knows where down there and the nurse is getting all glassy-eyed over the young guy who came in last week? Also why the emphasis on the "HE?"

Now **HE** was nice looking.

Okay, lady. I get that I am no Brad Pitt and maybe what you're dealing with down there is half the usual package you typically deal with BUT I AM A MAN WITH FEELINGS, GODDAMNIT. Well, no feelings in my loins or general pelvic area, but whatever.

*Now **HE** was nice looking. Not like Quasimodo Minidick over here.*

Right then I knew that confidentiality rules and professionalism fly right out the window if penises are involved and, sadly, that I was being compared to other guys while being flayed dong-side-up on the table. I assumed there was some sort of weird office pool going on in the urology office's kitchen and whoever got the square matching 4-inches length and 2-inches girth was about to be the big winner on the day.

There were a few more moments of that tugging sensation on the left side of my body, but I was busy hating myself for agreeing to undergo this entire process, so I did not really notice. One thing that was weird was that the tugging feeling felt like it was also coming from my butthole. I am not sure of the complete physiology of the male species, but I'm pretty positive that the testicles are not directly linked to the adjacent butthole, so I'm not quite clear on the connection there. Technically, they are only separated by a few inches so it is *possible* a little line connects them together. It would be cool if they were linked by two empty cans connected with a string so they could talk to each other.

> **Butthole** *[holding can up]*: Testicles, Testicles. This is Butt. Are you there, Testicles? Over.
>
> **Testicles:** We are here. Just hanging out. Over.
>
> **Doctor:** WHAT IN THE HELL.
>
> **Me:** Oh. Was I saying that out loud?

Then, the doctor said one of the most disturbing things I have ever heard in my life:

> **Doctor:** You may see some smoke.

Wait. What?

Smoke?

> **Me:** This is a doctor's office. I thought you couldn't smoke in here.

> **Doctor:** We are cauterizing you. Sometimes there is smoke.

> **Me:** Oh.

> **Doctor:** And we can smoke if we want. We're doctors.

I was really starting to not like these people.

Then I heard a sizzle.

A SIZZLE.

A SIZZLE FROM MY CROTCH.

It sounded like the doctor was making a teeny tiny piece of bacon. Just a little *'ssss'* sound coming out from between my legs. I glanced down because, although I couldn't feel it happening, the idea that there was crotch-bacon cooking was just too enticing to miss.

I looked towards my pelvis and there was a small mushroom cloud billowing out of my balls.

It was as if a microscopic nuclear bomb had been dropped on my right nut.

I sat transfixed, like an early settler seeing smoke signals on the horizon and realizing my chuck wagon was about to be attacked. The puff rose a foot or so, and then curled up and drifted away. As I watched my genitalia undergo the equivalent of a napalm attack, there was a second *'ssss'* sound as the doctor cauterized the same spot again, producing another little blast of smoke.

The smell was not good.

I have always heard that burning hair is probably the worst smell on the planet, but I'm going out on a limb here and claiming that burning balls are a close second. On a related note, I will not be grilling sausages for a while because I think the PTSD will be overwhelming.

The doctor and the nurse switched places and he repeated the cauterization on the other side. I felt like I was watching a flea circus re-enactment of *Apocalypse Now*. Miniature helicopters blasting over the horizon and launching their attacks on my testicles. I did not, however, love the smell of fire-grilled nuts in the morning (which, of course, I said in my head in my best Robert Duvall impression).

He put the flamethrower down, and after a few more random tugs he had sewn me up. I looked down to see only two stitches in each of my testicles. This surprised me because I figured with the amount of tugging, cutting, and volcanic eruptions that were happening it would have looked like Frankenstein's monster down there.

Nope. Just two tiny stitches. As if my groin got into a bar fight with a dwarf and all the little bastard had to attack me with were miniature bottles of Schnapps that he smashed on the bar.

> **Doctor:** You're done. Those stitches will dissolve in about ten days. You can get dressed and we will see you back here when you bring your final sample.

> **Me:** My what?

> **Doctor:** Your final sample. You need to ejaculate 25 times and bring in the 26th sample. They should have told you that in the consultation.

Ah, right. I had forgotten about that. I was so wrapped up thinking about shooting blasts of air out the end of my penis like a miniature leaf-blower that I had forgotten about the sample.

Me: Right.

He shook my hand, told me that there would be a prescription for painkillers at the front desk, and exited the room with the nurse. I assumed they were off to go check to see who had won the office pool.

I put on my jockstrap, gingerly pulled on my pants — taking extra care to stay as far away from the war zone as possible — and exited the office. I retrieved my glorious prescription for Vicodin from Marge, the office receptionist, who also handed me a tiny cup. She could only do this with one hand because her other hand was filled with $20 bills so looks like she won the office pool.

The cup she handed me was to hold #26.

Let the games begin.

Chapter 5

The AfterMATH (Whacks On, Whacks Off)

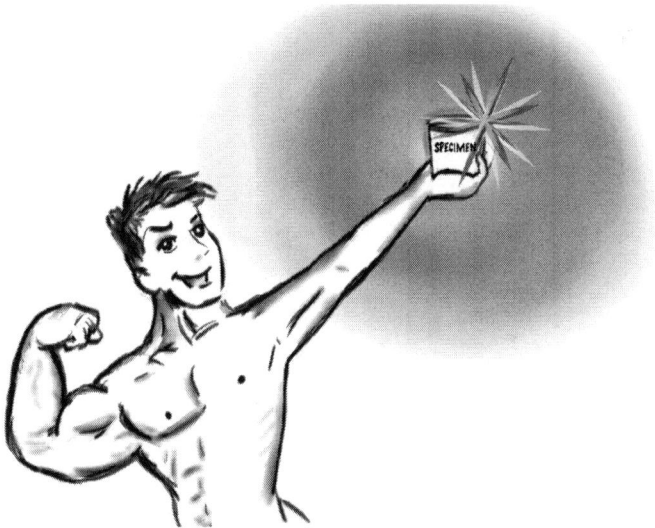

My phone keeps ringing with strange kids calling to wish me a Happy Father's Day. I should have saved the receipt on this vasectomy.

Day 20

Aside from the dull pain I have in my groin and the constant need to put something cold on my lap, this experience has not been nearly as bad as I had thought it was going to be. When you factor in the required bed rest and the Vicodin, it is actually a lot like being on vacation. That is, if, on the first day of vacation a doctor cut upon your genitals. If you can get past that, then yep, this is just like a vacation.

I have been using bags of frozen peas instead of ice on my crotch. The peas do a better job conforming to the lumpiness of a man's groin region and are also a great source of riboflavin and dietary fiber. I have been sitting in pajama pants because they are loose fitting and comfy and also I am not really out to impress anyone right now in the leisurewear category.

When Marge handed me the little cup for my 26th sample at the urologist's office, she said that she would see me in a couple of months. I asked why and she said, "It usually takes men eight weeks to get to the 26th sample."

Eight weeks?

That seems like an excessively long time.

I think I can really crush that out once my man-parts feel good enough to juggle them around again. Since we won't know if the operation actually "took" until we get the results from the sample, it looks like I'm on manual duty for numbers one through twenty-five. I am exhausted just thinking about it. On the bright side, my right arm is going to be massive and I can probably knock down a few pounds since I really put a lot of effort into jerkin' the gherkin and my heart rate rises very easily.

Eight weeks to get to number 26, though, seems like overkill.

CHALLENGE ACCEPTED.

Honestly, this should be its own game show or, at the very least, an immunity challenge on *Survivor*.

Jeff Probst: Men, you will need to produce 26 samples of-

Me: DONE. [clicks lever to raise team flag]

I think the only problems I'm going to have are (a) keeping this interesting because taking things into your own hands 26 straight times may get a bit monotonous and (b) keeping count. I already asked my wife and my original idea of keeping a tally by making large charcoal marks on the shower wall (like a prisoner marking his days of captivity) has been discouraged. This is mainly because she did not realize that masturbation was a shower activity. Right now she is in the middle of throwing out all our bars of soap.

I will ponder the method of keeping track later because I just came up with a great idea on how to keep myself interested in continually performing self-abuse. That sounds weird now that I've written it down. I mean, there is only so much porn someone can watch. I know this because I once took two weeks off from work, stayed home by myself, and reached the end of all the Internet porn by day three.

So I think what I'll do is just draw a face on the side of my hand. Like Señor Wences. I will have to rename it to Señorita Wences, though, because — even though I'm comfortable in my sexuality — I am not sure how my penis will react to a hand with a mustache on it heading towards him.

I could also draw faces on both hands. OOOH. My left hand will be the slutty one, Mistress Dangerpalm, and my right hand will be the prude one named Dorothy Lipslicker. It will be a physical embodiment of that saying, "Lefty Loosey, Righty Tighty." To make it even more interesting, I could just sit there and let my hands go at each other for a while first.

I like to watch.

Okay, so my wife just came in and saw my two hands kissing each other while I made smooching noises. I have also been advised that she is now rationing my Vicodin.

Mistress Dangerpalm is not happy about this.

Day 21

The idea hit me last night.

Actually, I had several ideas hit me last night. Most of them involved unicorns and my ability to speak Klingon. I don't think my wife's plan on rationing the Vicodin is working.

My idea was on how to keep track of my masturbatory sessions. Ready, Diary? You ready?

Two words:

ADVENT CALENDAR.

Bam.

We are approaching the holidays, right? I have to count up to 26 right?

There are 25 doors in an Advent calendar. As an added bonus, each door HAS CHOCOLATE BEHIND IT.

I cannot think of a more delicious way to buff my banana.

As a side note, my pain is slowly subsiding and I can walk around without much of an issue. My boss asked if I would be coming back to work soon but I think I'll milk it (not related to the above conversation) and see if I can get a free couple more days out of this. Using the terms "grapefruit sized" and "seepage" during the conversation should be good for scoring me at least three extra days. This might even get me out of actually talking to my boss for a while because no one wants to be on the receiving side of that conversation.

Okay, I'm going to head out and get an Advent calendar.

This is going to be awesome.

Day 22

Well, the Advent calendar was a terrible idea.

I went out to the local bookstore and grabbed one of their Advent calendars near the checkout counter. On the back of the calendar, there is a giant graphic showing you what is hidden inside the doors.

ALL PICTURES OF CHILDREN AND SANTA.

I forgot all about the pictures inside.

I do not want to find myself fiddling my flesh flute and then opening an Advent calendar door to find — BAM — a little girl and boy holding a puppy smiling back at me.

"HEY, WE KNOW WHAT YOU JUST DID YOU DISGUSTING MAN."

"SIR, PLEASE WASH YOUR HANDS BEFORE EATING THAT CHOCOLATE."

Dammit.

Therefore, I have decided I am just going to make my own calendar. The benefit of this is that now I can choose the kind of chocolate I get to eat instead of Hansel and Gretel over there handing me some cut-rate milk chocolate made in China that probably has metal shavings in it.

I am going with the *3 Musketeers* bar. I love love love me some *3 Musketeers.*

Flog my log? *3 Musketeers* bar.

Paddle the pickle? *3 Musketeers* bar.

Bop the bishop? *3 Musketeers* bar.

This is genius. Genius.

But that is a lot of candy. Even for an expert candy eater like me. I have a really high metabolic rate so I am usually not that worried about what I put into my body unless it came from the adult store on Main Street. When your wife comes home with a brown bag from an erotic toy store and a big bottle of ibuprofen, you can plan on very bad things happening.

Nevertheless, 25 candy bars is still a lot of candy. So, I went and calculated what additional damage this will do to my cholesterol-riddled body.

A full-size *3 Musketeers* has 260 calories. *Gadzooks*. I think that is a bit too much. 260 calories would sit around in my body for years. I hate cardio. I don't even like walking to my car.

A *3 Musketeers* miniature bar, though, only has 78 calories.

Okay, that's better. I'd be able to burn off the calories from a miniature three times faster than if I ate a full-sized bar so that would only take, say, four months. I could maybe burn it off in just two months if it's rerun season and I find motivation to get off the couch.

I have decided, then, to go with the miniature bars for the majority of my bologna-beating sessions. However, I am totally treating myself after #26 and going with the full-size bar because I'm an adult, dammit, and I can have a full-size candy bar if my wife says I can.

Okay. Let's do some math here. Kids, if you're reading this, stay in school. Math will someday come in handy; even if it is only for calculating your caloric intake from eating candy bars that you give yourself as an award for masturbating.

The more you know.

Here goes.

(25 x 78) + 260 = 2210 total calories ingested.

Okay, that isn't as bad as I first thought. I usually eat that in one sitting at the Chinese buffet. Maybe twice that amount if the buffet has pizza. Half of that if they don't have egg rolls.

I then Googled how many average calories are burned during sexual activity. I am assuming here that masturbation can be considered "sexual activity." However, if masturbation cannot be counted as sexual activity, then I may actually still be a virgin.

The results of this search provided me with a value of six to seven calories per minute of sexual activity. I also checked the "images" search results for "calories burned during sex" and, long story short, I lost three hours of my life looking at pictures of people having sex on yoga mats.

I added the seven-calorie/minute value into my equation and used my typical "time to completion" value to come up with how many calories I would burn each time I whacked my mole.

7 calories x 30-seconds to finish = 3.5 calories burned per session.

Okay, that sucks. If I could get myself to last any longer than 30 seconds, I would be able to burn off these candy bars at a much higher rate. Sadly, that saying, "If you want something done right, do it yourself" is also valid for doing yourself. As such, I have honed this entire procedure down to an exact science. I'm so good that I can finish myself off during a commercial break of *American Idol* and still have two minutes left over to get a snack before Ryan Seacrest starts being annoying again.

After thinking about this for a while, I decided to add another half-calorie for the effort it would then take me to go get a tissue/sock/stuffed animal to clean everything up. Then another half-calorie for actually doing the cleaning and another half-calorie for the 20 seconds of this that I'd spend dry-heaving. This brings me up to a grand total of five calories I'd burn off per plank-yank.

In the end, I ended up with this as a result:

5 calories x 25 salami slaps = 125 total calories burned.

In the end, I will be taking in 2210 calories from the *3 Musketeers*, and burning off 125.

I will be fat, but at least I will be satisfied.

Crap. Saying "satisfied" makes me want to redo all of this but with a *Snickers* instead.

Day 25

The good news is that the pain in my Golden Globes has subsided tremendously.

The bad news is the pain has subsided enough for me that I felt well enough to go back to work today.

It is not that I don't like working, it's just that I really despise it. I work in the computer industry, so most of my day is spent pretending that I know what I am doing. Sometimes I think it would take less effort to try to *do* the actual work instead of creating an elaborate façade to make it appear that I am working.

It has been roughly a week since the procedure and I am now officially out of painkillers. I am pretty bummed about this because I'm still holding off on starting the process of creating those samples. I do not want to accidentally bang my hand into something down there that is still healing and spend the next month in a full-body cast.

My stitches are still there on both sides, but will probably be gone soon. I cannot wait for this to happen because things in the southland get itchy occasionally and the self-restraint to not scratch the bejeezus out of them is turning out to be a difficult effort. Men spend roughly 75% of their day with their hands on their crotch. All this time is spent adjusting, moving, readjusting, drawing faces on their penis, scratching, pushing everything back between their legs while pretending they are a woman for a minute, and adjusting again. Refraining from all of this is killing me. I just hate the thought of popping a stitch and having all my guts exit one of my testicles, like when Hooper cuts open the tiger shark in *Jaws* and a Louisiana license plate spills out.

The guys at work, though, have been weird. They know why I was out but seem afraid to talk to me about it. I, on the other hand, wanted to tell everyone, which is why I wore my "Ask Me About My Vasectomy" t-shirt.

I think the guys are afraid of what I am going to say if they question me, though.

Coworker: So, how was it?

Me: It wasn't bad until they started doing it. Then it was basically a seven-hour marathon of watching a groin-only reboot of *The Texas Chainsaw Massacre* and felt like Muhammad Ali was treating my sack like a speed bag.

Maybe it's best that no one asked me about it. I have enough enemies at work already.

Day 26

Nothing really to report today other than my sack is still itchy, so to keep my mind occupied I have decided to see how many words I can make out of the word "Vasectomy." According to the Internet, you can make 268 words out of the letters in "vasectomy" but I don't have that kind of time or attention span, so I'm only going to list out the ones that I thought were appropriate and related to the procedure or nuts or I thought were funny.

Some words you can make from the letters in "Vasectomy:" Toy, yams, sac, set, stem, scam, scat, oats, seam, team, taco, veto, come, cats, came, mast, coma, meat, cast, mate, mayo, cave, vast, mosey, mateys, yeast, cameo, octaves, mascot and steamy.

If I think about it, I could probably come up with a good short story using some of those. At the very least, I could maybe come up with a decent paragraph.

My mate no longer wanted my meat mayo in her steamy taco. "Stem those yams or else scat," she said. What a scam. I wanted to veto, but I also wanted to continue to cast my mascot into her yeast moat. Taking one for the team, and risking a coma, my oats became tame. My voice is now three octaves higher. At least now I can set my toy in her vast cave without worrying if my sac mateys will make a cameo.

That was disturbing. I just pulled out the old pamphlet and there is nothing in there about mental instability as a potential side effect from the vasectomy.

I think I need to find something else to keep me busy.

Day 27

I was just looking through my desk drawer and found a note that my daughter wrote for me last year. Finding old things from your kids should not come as a surprise, Diary, because I'm a parent. Rule #86 in the Parenting Code clearly states, "All parents must keep everything a child has made since the beginning of time forever and ever. Items must either be stored in a folder or taped to a refrigerator." The housing market benefits from this because the majority of parents looking for a house simply need more storage room for arts and crafts or a kitchen big enough to hold multiple refrigerators.

I read the letter and decided it had to be entered in this journal.

Dear Dad,

I love you so much. You make me laugh and giggle every day. Even though you're short and have glasses, you're still very smart and the #1 dad in the universe.

You know why? You help me on my homework, you practice soccer with me, and you take all of us on vacation.

Remember when we won first place in bowling? We had that in common. We have another thing in common. We love Break-n-Bakes. You are special to me because you love me no matter what.

Hope this day is special.

Love,

Payton

Well, honey, it wasn't special before, but that changed after I found this letter. I particularly like the, "Even though you're short and have glasses," line. Well played.

For reference here, a "Break-n-Bake" is a store-bought cookie batter, already made. You just break off the squares and cook them and — bingo — you have cookies. It is a miracle of evolution.

This was a great reminder of how awesome kids can be. It's also a great reminder that I share a love of cookies with my children. Now I'm wondering if it would have been worth having another child just so I could have an excuse to eat more cookies.

I'm off to find the kids, Diary. Eating cookies seems like a great way to kill time while I'm waiting for these damn stitches to fall out.

Day 28

THEY'RE GONE!

I got out of the shower this morning, and my stitches had finally disappeared!

Of course, I then spent the next hour feeling my stitch-less self because it has been almost two weeks where my dangly bits did not feel like they were wrapped in barbed wire. Unfortunately, because I've had stitches in there, I have been unable to perform my manscaping duties so essentially my kiwis felt like, well, kiwis. Actually, the fuzz had grown past the soft-and-fluffy kiwi stage and was approaching a wire hairbrush level of coarseness. My crotch looked like two baby hedgehogs sharing a cocktail frank.

Then I noticed the scars.

If I rotate each of my grapes up a little bit, I can see a small quarter-inch long scar on the outside of them. The scar on Mr. Righty has healed quite nicely. It is in the shape of a smile and, honestly, he brightened my day a little bit. It got even better when I dotted two eyes and a nose above it. He looked so happy to not have his mouth sewn shut anymore.

The left side, though. What in the actual hell happened to you, Mr. Lefty?

The scar on my left testicle (leftsicle?) looked like Elvis doing that thing he always did with his top lip and trying to frown at the same time while eating a lemon. It was crooked and lumpy. The result was one angry looking left nut.

So now I have one happy ball and one angry ball. It is like those two comedy/tragedy drama masks but the masks are being worn by my beanbags.

On the bright side, though, now I can get back to shaving these things. Then I can start working on abusing myself in order to get those samples done. I should probably stop drawing happy/sad faces on my privates and maybe start carb-loading.

Day 29

It happened.

I wish to god it did not, but it happened nonetheless.

I went into the shower this morning with my razor in hand, intent on clearing my South American rainforest.

Harvesting the crops.

Mowing the lawn.

Weeding my lower garden.

I was going to be shaving my groin stubble, just for clarification here.

I started in. There was roughly two weeks' worth of overgrowth down there, but not enough that I needed to break out the beard trimmer again. Instead, I went straight at myself with my razor.

On the first swipe, I felt it.

nick

NOOOOOOOOOOOOOOOOOOOOO!!

I had, on the very first swipe of the blade, cut my nut. I totally nick-nacked my paddywhack. I thought there could be no worse feeling than having my testicle injected with a hypodermic needle but, nope, I was wrong. Snagging yourself with a razor blade on the side of your ball tops that.

The culprit was that stupid, mangled, frowny-lemon faced-Elvis-scar on my left side. What was once an area that could be easily traversed is now a patch of rough terrain that requires the use of four-wheel drive to get over. Now that I think of it, that would actually be a funny Land Rover commercial.

nick

The horror that came with the realization of what I had just done was terrifying. When the razor caught, I did that reflexive little suck-up of my breath with that *'ffttt'* noise, and the razor dropped from my hands, clanking on the shower floor below. I did NOT want to look down.

What if I was bleeding?

What if my entire nut was gone?

How would I explain this to the 9-1-1 operator?

911: 9–1–1. What is your emergency?

Me: MY GOD!! THE BLOOD!!!

911: Sir, you'll need to calm down. What's the problem, sir?

Me: THE TWINS. I'VE...DONE SOMETHING...HORRIBLE TO THE TWINS...

911: Sir-

Me: MY BABIEEEES

911: Sir. Please calm down and explain your situation.

Me: What was I thinking?! Three blades?! THREE?!?

911: Sir, you said "twins." Are your children hurt, sir?

Me: Yes. Wait, no. Not "twins" as in "kids." My balls. I almost cut off a nut while shaving. PLEASE HURRY.

911: Uh...

Me: WAIT. Okay, okay. I'm good. I washed off the apricot soap scrub with active botanicals that I used instead of shaving cream and it turns out that I just scraped it. It's not bleeding too badly.

911: Are you talking about cutting your testicle while shaving?

Me: Yeah. Phew. Okay. A small *Dora the Explorer* bandage should cover it. I *do* have a question, though. Before the paramedics arrive, should I finish shaving the nut or just leave everything half-done?

911:

Me: Hello?

Thankfully, it wasn't nearly as bad as I had imagined. I made a mental note, at that moment, to be especially careful around the boys when taking them to the barbershop from this point forward. The terrain is fairly treacherous now thanks to my misshapen vasectomy scars and I will always need to proceed with extreme caution.

I am seriously pitching this to Land Rover, though. This would make an amazing 30-second spot.

Day 31

A
All
All je
All jerk
All jerk an
All jerk and n
All jerk and no p
All jerk and no pla
All jerk and no play m
All jerk and no play mak
All jerk and no play makes
All jerk and no play makes Ro
All jerk and no play makes Rod a
All jerk and no play makes Rod a du
All jerk and no play makes Rod a dull
All jerk and no play makes Rod a dull boy.

Well, it's apparent that whittling down the days of my Advent calendar by whittling my own wood is seriously taking a toll on my mind and spirit.

It's also apparent that I really need to find myself a hobby. Holy shit.

Day 32

Captain's Log: Stardate something something something.

I am now up to nine candy bars.

Without getting into the gory details, Diary, I can tell you that getting these samples done is not as easy as you would think. The big problem I am having is that I'm not always in the mood for chocolate. I'm also not always in the mood for pounding my flounder, either. I think there is a big difference in knowing I *have* to do this versus me thinking it's something fun to do.

I am guessing this is how professional athletes feel. A game is enjoyable when you're just playing for fun but being *required* to play turns it into a chore and that takes a lot of the joy out of it. Then again, pro athletes are all getting million-dollar salaries, so they can suck it up and play. Me? I'm getting a bunch of tiny candy bars and maybe type 2 diabetes. Huge difference. HUGE.

A few times, I have paddled my panda without going for the candy bar reward. Then other times I'll think, "I could go for some chocolate" and go eat a few bars in one sitting, thinking I will make up for it later. This turned out to be a fun conversation when my wife left to go shopping and came back 30 minutes later to find three candy bar wrappers in the trash. She assumed that as soon as she walked out the door I was running around with my underwear at my ankles, covering my nether-regions in Vaseline and just going to town on myself.

Nope. I just had a hankering for some nougat.

On a side note, the razor incident is now in my rear-view mirror and I can see that things in my southern territories are settling quite nicely. The scars on my marbles are actually starting to flatten out, so manscaping efforts *should* be a little easier now. Just to be sure, though, I am using a single blade razor from this point forward. Two blades mean twice the damage if something goes wrong and I'm all about minimizing risk when it comes to possibly shearing off my cojones.

I should probably put you down, Diary, and get to work on these other 16 samples. I wish I could do the multiple-orgasm thing that women can supposedly do. Now that I'm thinking about that, the visual of turning myself into a human Gatling gun would probably work well in the porn adaptation of *Terminator.*

Terminator [opening door]: Sarah Conner?

Sarah Conner: Yes?

Terminator: [kicks down door, opens coat and starts machine-gun shooting from the hip]

Sarah: MY EYE! IT STINGS!

I'd watch that.

If I could do that then I'd probably be done by now, for sure. Sitting around comfortably with a belly full of chocolate, getting insulin injections.

A man can dream.

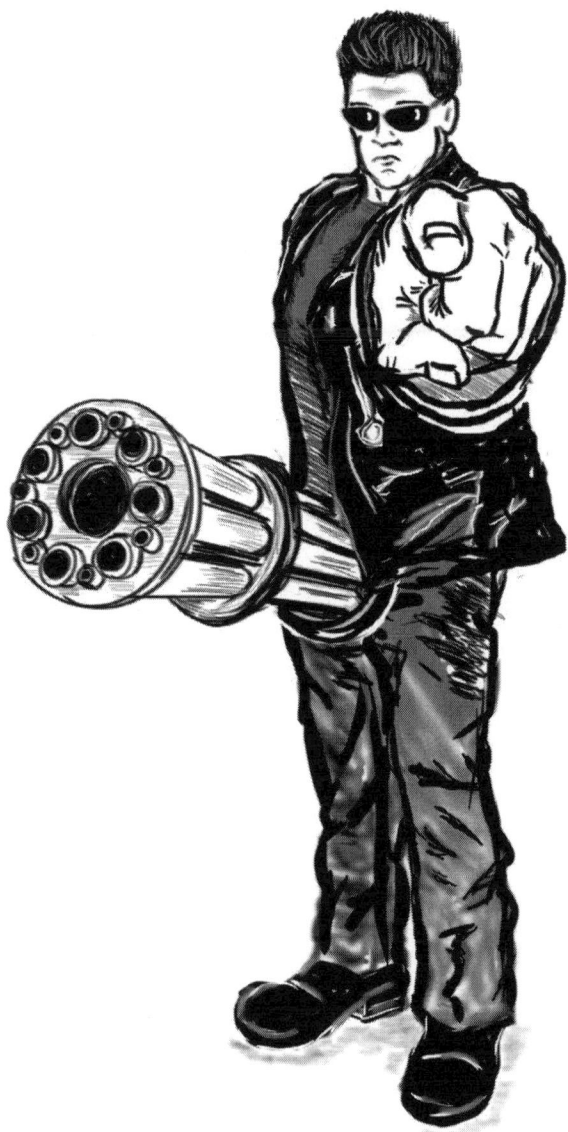

Day 35

Every so often, there is a need for me to validate the entire process of getting a vasectomy. Yesterday was one of those days, and the validation came in the form of flushable wipes.

Flushable wipes.

We have a bathroom on the far side of the house that is part of a fairly new addition. The sewer pipe leading from the shower/toilet/sink in that bathroom runs right through my basement and is about a foot above my head when I'm standing below it.

When my first child was potty training, we found a wonderful new product called the "flushable wipe." The flushable wipe was a godsend because anyone who has ever cleaned off a kid's ass after they crapped into a diaper knows that it is probably about as close to smelling death as you can get. Cleaning it up, though, is actually like staring Death itself right in the face. There is a horrific stench and sometimes it's squishy and sometimes IT IS UP THE CHILD'S BACK OMG HOW DID THAT HAPPEN and, in those moments, you just want to teach your kid to go poop and pee outside like the dog does.

Then came the miracle of flushable wipes.

When your kid poops, you put him on the changing table, open his diaper and then focus on suppressing your gag reflex while trying not to throw up all over your own child. Then you reach over, pull out one of these magical flushable wipes, wipe his disgusting crap-coated bum, throw the wipe into the toilet and just flush it away. VOILA! There is no Diaper Genie, bags or lingering stink unless you got some poo on your hand. Then you want to die a thousand times over. The flushable wipe, however, is gone. Everything just magically goes down the toilet and is gone forever and ever until the toilet water reappears as drinking water from your faucet after undergoing sewage treatment. Okay, I am never drinking water ever again.

The poop, pee, and wipes, though, are thankfully no longer in your house. They are out of sight and out of mind.

Usually.

Yesterday, the shower and toilet in our new bathroom both started backing up. I can tell you that there is nothing like seeing poop water backing up into your shower to make you wish it were legal to poop straight into the sewer grates on the street, or at least be able to do it without being yelled at by the neighbors again.

My father's side of the family is made up entirely of carpenters and construction workers. I, personally, cannot hammer a nail into a wall without something exploding or catching on fire, but I have watched enough to pick up a few handy tricks. One of these things was being able to check a pipe to pinpoint where a clog could possibly be. I headed down to the basement to find the source of the backup, but not before my wife gave me a fire extinguisher because she's been around enough of my home improvement projects to know better.

I found the 4" PVC sewer pipe leading from the bathroom and tapped on it. The noise that came back indicated that it was completely clogged.

No big deal. All I had to do was unscrew the fitting on the side of the pipe and snake down to where the clog was. Easy peasy. My wife stood behind me and watched as I climbed up on a chair, wrench in hand, and started to unscrew the cleanout pipe fitting in front of me.

About a quarter of a turn in, the fitting came loose and *exploded* off the pipe. It pegged me straight in the forehead and bounced off somewhere into the basement.

Behind it, a thousand pressurized gallons of backed-up shower water and poop and pee gushed directly into my face. I tried to put my hands over the 4-inch hole once occupied by the fitting, but all it did was get poop and pee and shower water all over my hands and now on our laundry.

It was like that scene in *Flashdance* but instead of Jennifer Beals being provocatively splashed with water, it was me in an AC/DC t-shirt drowning in a never-ending waterfall of raw sewage. I turned my face to look at my wife who was running out of the way and laughing hysterically.

It's so important to have the support of your loved ones.

The deluge seemed to go on forever. When it finally subsided, we had a small, stinky ocean in our basement, and I also probably had a bad case of dysentery. I stepped down from the chair, found the pipe fitting half-submerged in sludge, screwed it back in, and asked my wife if she could hand me a towel after she was done crying from laughter. I dried off, took a 37-hour shower under scalding water, and called a plumber to clear the clog.

Flushable wipes.

The clog was downstream, caused by approximately 1,000 flushable wipes. According to the plumber, flushable wipes are called "flushable" because they are small enough to go down the toilet. They do not dissolve like toilet paper but, instead, can cause a clog in your plumbing that will eventually lead to you requiring a tetanus shot and being on really strong antibiotics just for precaution.

I write this, my dearest Diary, as another example of why I have gone through this vasectomy torture. I am not saying I would ever trade in my children, but I certainly know how I'd choose between not having a new baby and potentially being covered in little brown canoes someday.

Day 40

8:45 AM

DONE.

I'm done I'm done I'm done.

As I write this, I am sitting here enjoying the fruits of my labor: the full-size *3 Musketeers* bar. Next to me, on this desk, is a small container holding the Holy Grail of the vasectomy procedure:

Sample #26.

It's actually kind of gross, now that I am thinking about it. I am not sure what to do with it. I'm certainly not putting it in the fridge next to the yogurt, that's for damn sure.

The effort required to get that stupid sample into that tiny container was nothing to laugh at, let me tell you. I didn't really think of what I needed to do until I'd actually started doing it. In hindsight, though, I am not sure I could do anything differently because a man's anatomy only works one way.

I think.

I went upstairs to my bedroom this morning, cup in hand, to go get 'er done. I sat on my bed and brought up the usual offerings of late-night Cinemax On-Demand but I had pretty much watched all of it trying to get through numbers one through twenty-five. I finally settled on the Home Shopping Network because Rachael Ray was there talking about a new cookbook.

To whoever reads this diary: please do not judge me.

I was lying there, just listening to Rachael's melodious voice talking about things that were "delish" and saying "e-v-o-o" when I realized that my little Mount Vesuvius was about to rain down on Pompeii. In this analogy, I am playing the role of Pompeii.

I grabbed the cup, took the lid off, and then realized my volcano was pointing *up*. When a man's love-volcano is about to erupt it points to the sky because it is easier to sacrifice virgins that way, I suppose. *It's science.* However, this posed an interesting question:

HOW WAS I GOING TO GET THE SAMPLE INTO THE CUP?

I tried to force-bend it down a little bit so that gravity could take over, but that was pretty hurty and I did not want to break him. I leaned him to the right but that was also a little hurty and also I did not want anything to overshoot and possibly land on my side of the bed. I leaned it to the left because I didn't care if anything got on my wife's side of the bed, but I could still not get the angle right.

I flipped over onto my stomach but that was even more awkward. Trying to keep everything going with one hand, holding the sample cup in the other, and trying to keep my balance on the mattress with only my toes and forehead touching the bed. I'm pretty sure that maintaining this position is a required skill for passing Navy Seals training.

I had to stand up.

Rachael Ray was already wrapping up her sales pitch, so I was quickly running out of time. With my little bomb reaching critical mass, I stood up and bent over as far as I could. This only got my little love missile to a parallel angle to the ground and, in my current yoga position, horrifyingly aimed directly at my face. With as much balance as I could muster, I forced him a little towards the ground with my working hand and held the cup in the other.

I have seen Cirque de Soleil shows with less acrobatic displays.

It worked. I was able to get 95% of sample #26 into the cup. The other 5% was just collateral damage and easily cleaned up using my wife's slippers.

All my pain, sweat, callouses, and tears paid off.

I stood up, listening to my back crack roughly 300 times and screwed the cap on the sample container. I picked up the phone and called the urologist's office.

> **Marge:** Urology Specialists. How can I help you?
>
> **Me:** Hi, this is Rodney Lacroix. I had a vasectomy there about a month ago.
>
> **Marge:** Yes, Rodney. What can I do for you?
>
> **Me:** The squirrel is in the nest.
>
> **Marge:** Um. Excuse me?
>
> **Me:** The chicken is in the coop. The yogurt is in the vegan section.
>
> **Marge:** Are you having a seizure?
>
> **Me:** I have my 26th sample.
>
> **Marge:** Okay. Drop it off anytime.

Marge would make a terrible spy.

I am heading down there in a little while to say goodbye to #26 and wish him well in all his testing. I should know the results in a few days so I am going to take some time off here, Diary, to help my arms, hand, and penis recover from the beatings. In the meantime, I'm going to savor this big candy bar before I head over there to drop it off.

That reminds me. I did not wash my hands after. I may go throw up.

4:30 PM

Well, that was fun.

After I put this diary down earlier, I finished my candy bar, grabbed #26 and headed downstairs. I opened the kitchen cabinet, found a small paper bag and placed it inside. I figured people were not just walking into the place with a clear cup of their own DNA sloshing around like it was a tiny iced mocha latte.

"Daddy, what's this?"

I turned to see my daughter holding the paper bag, about to open it and look inside.

CHRIST ON A CRACKER!

I leaped for it like I was trying to take a bullet for her. I snatched the bag from her tiny little hands, and she immediately started to cry. The thought, "Don't cry over spilled milk" crossed my mind and I felt myself throw up in my mouth a little bit.

Wife: It's something daddy has to take to the doctor.

Nice save.

I got to the urologist's office and was second in line waiting for the receptionist. Everyone in the waiting room seemed to be looking at me as I stood there holding the paper bag. I could see them trying to figure out if it was pee in there or *the other stuff* because they'd look at the bag, then at me, then at the bag, then at me. In my head, I knew they were thinking, *"He's got goo."*

I could feel them sizing it up by gauging the amount of blood rushing to my face. I just wanted to throw the bag through the opening in the receptionist's window like it was a can of teargas and just get the hell out of there.

A man stepped into the office and got in line behind me. As I glanced back, I saw that he, too, was holding a bag. His paper bag was the fancy kind like from Pier One or Crate and Barrel, with the little wire handles instead of the five-cent "mom gave me crackers and water again" bargain-store lunch bag I had crimped up in my tiny little hands. Like his #26 was better than mine.

Marge: NEXT!

I handed Marge my hobo-package and gave her my name. She then handed me back two more cups.

Wait. What?

Why was she giving me more cups? I did not recall anything about bringing in a #27 or #28 or anything. Maybe these were just souvenir cups, like the ones you get at Six Flags that come with free refills.

Thinking about that, I threw up in my mouth a little again.

Me: What are these for?

Marge: One is just in case we need another one for whatever reason, and the other cup is for the next sample that you'll have to bring to an independent lab.

Me: But...I'm so, so tired.

Marge: You'll hear from us in a couple of days.

Me: So tired.

Marge [*looking past me now*]: NEXT.

Me: DAMMIT MARGE I AM NOT A MASTURBATION MACHINE.

I turned and sauntered past Mr. Precocious-sperm and his fancy goo-bag. Then I stopped off at CVS on the way home and picked up two more *3 Musketeers* bars.

One for #27, and the other one just in case.

Chapter 6

The Vas Deferens Verdict

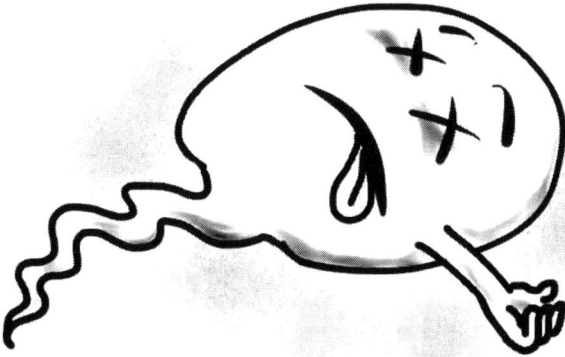

Just virus-scanned my computer and found three Trojans, which is weird because I have a vasectomy and don't need them.

Day 42

Negative.

I have often been called a negative person, but usually this is only by people who know me. Sometimes it is by people who do not know me. I can be a real asshole most times, so I see where that comes from.

But the call I got this morning was not about me, no. The call that came in was all about #26.

Nurse: Your test was negative.

Me: Give it to me straight. How long have I got?

Nurse: What?

Me: I'm dying, right? Wait. Which doctor's office is this?

It was the urologist's office. My sample came back as negative for any live baby-makers. The swimming pool was empty. The river had run dry. There was no more room at the inn.

I probably should not have turned that into a Bible reference.

Nurse: Your sample was negative.

Me: Really?

Nurse: *Very* negative. It was the meanest sample we have ever had to deal with. It was catcalling the other nurses and asked the lab technician if he had gotten his diploma via mail-order.

Me: Well, that explains why my kids can be such jerks.

I was very excited about the results, though, to say the least. That meant I did NOT have to go back to have the procedure looked at and could probably begin having sex again once I found someone who wanted to do it with me. Early projections had me getting to third base with someone within the next decade.

> **Nurse:** You will need to take your next sample to an independent lab.

Ugh. The other cups.

> **Nurse:** Make your appointment. Also, this sample can be no more than an hour old.

Oh. No pressure, thanks. One of my strengths is being able to play tug-of-war with the cyclops and then speed the resulting sperm sample across town in my Honda Civic. Piece of cake, lady.

I made the appointment after I got off the phone with her. Ironically, the lab is in the same hospital where my children were born. I tried to explain how this was funny to the person on the other end of the phone making the appointment but apparently she was related to Marge and did not really have time for any of my shenanigans. It's like urology receptionists have their own union and you can only get in if you have zero sense of humor.

My appointment for dropping off #27 is tomorrow morning. I had better go gas up the car and get a tune-up because the hospital is 45 minutes away from here. Dropping that thing off in under an hour is going to be close.

Maybe I can get a police escort. Or maybe I can just make the sample in the hospital parking lot.

I am going to scratch that last idea. Once I made a sample in a public parking lot and got a different kind of police escort.

Day 43

Forty-eight minutes. I got to the hospital in 48 minutes with #27. I would have gotten there sooner but I was stuck behind an old man in a Buick. Why is it that old people always drive Buicks and they all have to go 3 mph under the speed limit? It's as if they don't want to get where they're going. You would think that at their age they would want to get there as soon as possible so they can do what they need to do before they die. Boggles my mind.

I burst through the doors of the lab like I had been shot and was in need of a doctor in the emergency room screaming "I HAVE #27! I HAVE #27!" No one knew what I was talking about, obviously, but I was so exhausted from running up the eight steps of the lab that someone got me a sweet wheelchair and a glass of water.

I handed over #27 and was told it would be a couple of days before I hear the results. This ordeal is taking way longer than I thought it would. On the bright side, I am only on Day 43. According to Marge, the typical man wouldn't even be close to having his #26 ready by this point, so I'll just pat my back as an overachiever.

Okay, the patting kind of winded me a little bit. I'm glad I'm still sitting in this wheelchair.

Day 45

Dear Diary,

I would like to thank you for being here for me. For having an avenue to write in and talk about my thoughts and feelings and even the hallucinations I had while on Vicodin.

But now it is time we say goodbye.

Today, I found out that #27 was also a negative sample!! PRAISE JEEBUS IT WAS NEGATIVE! That's right, my darling Diary:

I'm free and clear, my friend.

The bullets have left the chamber.

My flying Elvis' have left the airplane.

My pool is full of dead swimmers.

My CIA intelligence is less than accurate.

My ballistic missile has been disarmed.

Scarlett Johansson is really hot.

I just needed to throw that one in there in the event she ever reads this diary. I just want her to know how I feel about her.

The term the nurse actually used when she called was "free and clear." I have always known my sperm was free because charging women for it just seems mean. However, this was the first time it was ever called "clear." Basically, she was telling me that there were no swimmers in the second sample, which means, officially, the vasectomy took.

Apparently, I still do have live things living around down there, but when it's "go time," they essentially run up the vas deferens and then – BAM – dead end. It's like that time I was in Florida trying to get to Universal Studios but my GPS kept giving me directions sending me into this alley that only had a dumpster at the end of it. In that analogy, I am the sperm, the alley is my vas deferens, and I guess my rental car is playing the part of my penis.

So there, sweet little Diary, is where this entire vasectomy story comes to a close. All things must come to an end, they say.

In this case, though, it all comes to a dead end.

Literally.

I'm sorry I woke up screaming, but I had a nightmare that I had my vasectomy reversed.

Epilogue – A Note from the Author

Today, my vasectomy is still holding strong, much like the kid from *The Little Dutch Boy* sticking his finger in the dike to save Holland from a flood. Okay, that is a terribly upsetting analogy. Maybe it is more like the Great Wall of China and how it held back tribes of northern invaders. Okay, that doesn't really make sense, either. I've got it. Let's call him "Warden Vasectomy" who runs the maximum-security Penile Penitentiary and he has a 100% success rate at stopping his most virile prisoners from escaping.

I may be overthinking this.

I have never regretted having my vasectomy done. I love my kids, for sure, but I certainly do not want to make any more of them. I am older now and tire much more easily. In addition, schools have changed to something called "Common Core Math" which requires you to add numbers by creating a complex algorithm using blocks and shapes and hieroglyphs. I refuse to have another child and have to go through helping THAT kid with Common Core math in six years.

So if I am keeping a tally here of pros and cons, I can come up with this:

PROS:

- No more children

- No more children = no more diapers/sleepless nights/poo under my fingernails

- Single men can have unprotected sex with anyone after they pass a 21-point inspection, blood test, and sign a non-disclosure agreement

- Married men can have unprotected sex with their spouse (representing a savings of up to $3.99 annually on condoms!)

- Women apparently dig a guy with a vasectomy

That last part probably should not be discounted.

I did a lot of Tweeting, posting and blogging about my vasectomy during the process. This is primarily because I'm an attention whore and, according to my family, "nothing is sacred" and "I have shamed them." However, I received a *lot* of responses from women about it. It seemed like the majority of women who read my posts would respond with things like, *"Wait. You can't get me pregnant? Pick me up at six."*

I quickly realized that a vasectomy was a potentially HUGE selling point for a guy looking to get dates with women. Obviously, if you're on Christian Mingle then a vasectomy is actually a turn-off because they require that the only birth-control members practice be celibacy, the rhythm method, or a combo of both (the latter can only be done through pants with John the Baptist's face printed on them).

CONS:

- I haven't seen my testicles in eight years

Honestly, I have no idea why this happens. Shortly after my vasectomy, my testicles decided to look around one day, realize they were no longer needed and just left town. Where they fled to, I have no idea. All they did was leave a note on my table saying "Heading out for cigarettes, back later. – Nuts."

I never saw them again.

I do not know if this is a common side effect of the vasectomy, but my yam bags are now officially AWOL. Every so often, when it is warm out, they will magically reappear and we will sit around and reminisce about the good old days when they would be around constantly. Then – boom – off they retreat to the inner workings of my abdomen. It is a little weird and embarrassing to no longer have visible giggleberries, but it's something I have learned to deal with. Luckily, my wife is fully aware there may or may not be a showing of the little guys and it is completely out of my control. I've bought tickets to several *Guns N' Roses* shows where Axl didn't even bother leaving his hotel so I know exactly how she feels.

Ladies, if you're with a man who's had the procedure done, cut him some slack and try not to say things like, "Where are your balls?" and "Did you have your nuts removed?" and "Are you a woman?" because it's not helping. Post-vasectomy balls have a mind of their own.

I hope you enjoyed my diary and hope you find it entertaining enough to share with friends, family, baby daddies, or anyone who would get a kick out of the stories. It is probably best not to share these tales with kids, though. I do not think children want to know how much punishment a man will endure to ensure that he does not make any more of them.

Be aware, though, that handing this to a man who has already had a vasectomy may bring about PTSD.

Post Testicle Stress Disorder.

It's probably a real thing.

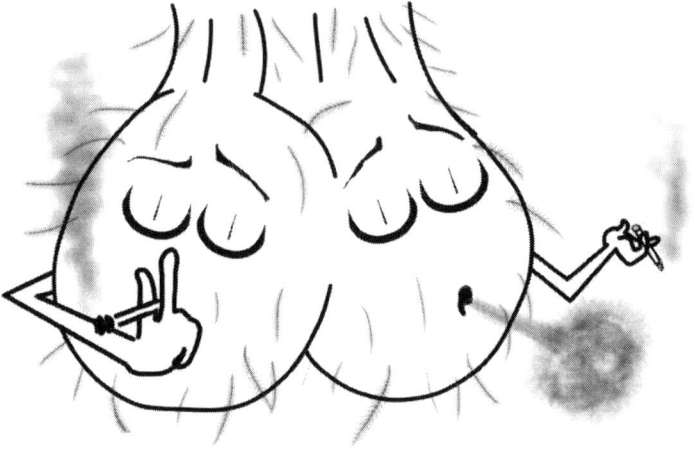

Glossary of Terms

Tes·ti·cle 'testək(ə)l/*noun*

Plural noun: testicles

Definition: Either of the two oval organs that produce sperm in men and other male mammals, enclosed in the scrotum behind the penis.

Synonyms: balls, nuts, deez nutz, nards, nads, gonads, boys, dangly bits, family jewels, grapes, cajones, stones, beanbags, huevos, sandbags, jingle bells, walnuts, rocks, sweetbreads, testes, bells, clappers, bollocks, slappers, bojangles, kiwis, crown jewels, knackers, privates, baubles, plums, ballbag, goolies, junk, naughty bits, spunk bunkers, berries, wedding tackle, scallops, marbles, targets, groin, itchy and scratchy, cream donuts, doo-dahs, scrotum, scrote, fruit basket, giblets, Mutt 'n' Jeff, nuggets, acorns, conkers, coin purse, chestnuts, the twins, wheelies, bullet bags, spuds, two veg, billiards, sperm banks, orbs, brains, agar jellies, baby sack, seed bag, beans, eggs, Ben Wahs, frozen exam, Jehovah's Witnesses

Mas·tur·bate 'mastər‚bāt/*verb*

Definition: Stimulate one's own genitals for sexual pleasure.

Synonyms (male only): bashing the candle, bleeding the weasel, bleedin the weed, buffing the banana, bopping the baloney, burping the worm, choking the chicken, cleaning your rifle, corking the bat, cranking the shank, cuffing the carrot, fisting your mister, flogging your dog, flogging the frog, flogging the hog, flogging the log, flute solo, jerkin' the gherkin, looping the mule, manual override, painting the pickle, pocket pinball, pocket pool, polishing the banister, polishing the rocket, pounding your flounder, pumping the python, roping the pony, spanking the monkey, teasing the weasel, tossing the turkey, walking the dog, whipping the willy, wonking your cronker, yanking the crank

About the Author

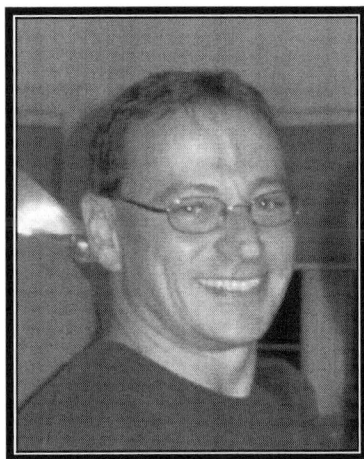

Rodney Lacroix is a devoted husband and father of two biological and two step-children. He resides in Southern New Hampshire where he splits time between his job and, well, all those kids. Rodney is a part-time comedian, full-time software engineer, reluctant soccer coach, and terrible guitar player.

He also hopes you enjoyed this book. If you'd like to read the other best-selling comedy books in his repertoire, you can find them on Amazon:

Things Go Wrong for Me – When Life Hands You Lemons, Add Vodka

Perhaps I've Said Too Much – A Great Big Book of Messing with People

Romantic as Hell – A Guide for the Romantically Challenged

You can also find him on Twitter as *@mooooooog35*, Facebook as *RodneyLacroixAuthor* and on his website, *RodneyLacroix.com.*

Acknowledgements

I would like to thank my wife, Kerri, my kids and step-kids (Payton, Cameron, Evan, and Ashlyn) and my friends and family for all of their continued support. I would also like to give a *special* additional shout-out to my children because they are pretty mad that I once again published a book I will not allow them to read until they've moved out of the house. I'm sorry, guys.

I would also like to thank the litany of people who helped edit and shape this book. In no particular order:

Cover Art: Houston Keys

Illustrations: Noreen Conway

Editors-at-Large: Ben Gott, Holly Hegler, Hilary L. Jastram, Joshua E. Smith, Amy Mayo, Brandi Hanton, Caroline Wright, Jennifer Parsons and Heather Rosen. If there are typos or Oxford commas or anything else they may have missed, please feel free to blame them.

Friends, Romans, Countrymen: Steve Gelder, Neal Veglio, Suzy Soro, Jenna McCarthy, Dave Womach, Alex Belisle

To anyone I forgot to mention but who contributed to the content herein, thank you. Also, please forgive me for excluding you here, but I am really old and can't remember anything without writing it down.

25554647R00077

Printed in Great Britain
by Amazon